MW01222537

DATE DUE

MAY 2 2 2015	

Mommy, Please Don't Listen To Them

DENISE F. LOEWEN

a little girls story about her fight for life.

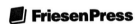 **FriesenPress**

Suite 300 – 852 Fort Street
Victoria, BC, Canada V8W 1H8
www.friesenpress.com

ISBN
978-1-4602-5108-9 (Hardcover)
978-1-4602-5109-6 (Paperback)
978-1-4602-5110-2 (eBook)

1. Family & Relationships, Children with Special Needs

Distributed to the trade by The Ingram Book Company

Be kind to all those you meet in this world. You never know when one day you may be walking your path in their shoes. How grateful you will be when good karma comes your way.

Table of Contents

I dedicate this book to my daughter, Trina Dawn, a beautiful angel who came to this Earth from Heaven and gave us 27 wonderful years of wisdom. She came to teach every one of us the true meaning of family and friendship. She made my family strong, kind, and grateful for every blessing, no matter how small. Trina, I am so very grateful for the time I had with you. I know that you are in a better place. I miss you so much. The void in my heart caused by losing your physical being cannot be filled by anything else here on this Earth. You have given me true love.

Thank You's

Thank you to Jackie, Trina's wonderful sister. Because of your love for Trina and coming back home, I could always take great care of her the way she deserved. You are the big sister that every little girl dreams about, and the best daughter a mother could ever have. Trina will float on your shoulder for eternity.

Thank you to Jonathon, Trina's big brother and knight in shining armour. Trina knew who she was choosing when she chose you to be her protector while she walked her path. With you beside her she had no fear. You have become an amazing young man and no mom could be prouder than I to have you as a son.

Thank you to Tom, Trina's brother-in-law. Thank you for spending so much time with Trina you always had a special way with her. She would cuddle with you for hours. When you feel like your not alone on the couch, well you know who is there with you.

Thank you to my brother Dean, Trina's uncle. Trina missed you before you even left the yard. It gives me peace of mind to know that Trina has you in Heaven with her. I can see the two of you playing basketball, just like you did with her on Earth.

Thank you to my niece Megan, Dean's daughter. What can I say Megan? Trina loved you so much. You were a little sister to her. You were in her thoughts every time she came out of a seizure. "Megan, Megan, Megan," would be her first words. I could not be prouder of you for being the beautiful person you are.

Thank you to Annabella, Pixie, and Kaleb. Auntie Trina loved you so much and your love for her made her want to be with you always. I know she will live on and on in your hearts.

Thank you to my dad, Trina's grandpa. It was because of your love for me that I was able to love and never give up. The strength that you showed us as children has been passed on in all of us. You were always there for me when I was scared. You were the best grandpa—your grandchildren have nothing but smiles when they think of you. Take care of my baby.

Thank you to every beautiful child who lived in our home. You brought the world to Trina. The love that you showed her will be with her forever. I know she smiles down on you and yours everyday.

Thank you to all my wonderful friends. Your love was always felt in our home. I thank you for understanding why I always chose to put Trinafirst, above everything else in this world and for not leaving me behind.

Denise F. Loewen

Thank you Kristen and Michelle. You held us together and became our ears and strength during our time of helplessness and sorrow.

Thank you to our family doctor, Dr. P. Yanko—or Uncle Yanko, as Trina called you. Without you in our lives, Trina's journey here on Earth would have been shortened. You saved her life and restored my faith and trust in the medical field over and over again. You are like a big brother to me. The crystal had a meaning like no other. Trina loved you so much.

Thank you to all of Trina's teachers. I can't say in words how grateful I am to you. You took my place while Trina was in school and kept her safe while she was not in my care. It was because of you that Trina loved each and every day of school. Martin, Trina never forgot you.

Thank you to Judy and Wayne. Because of you and your love our family was able to be by Trina's side during the hardest time of our lives.

Thank you, Tim. You will never know how grateful I am for that you were by Trina's side at the hospital. You gave me calm knowledge that I needed so deeply. The kindness and gentleness you showed Trina will never be forgotten.

Thank you, Dr. Takahashi. It was because you chose to listen to me and search for the truth that Trina was able to celebrate her 23 birthday. I will always remember how much you cared.

Prologue

I have written this book with love in memory of my daughter Trina. I was Trina's voice all her life. I hope to reach those who have a loved one who depends on their voice to keep them healthy and alive. It was her fight for life that made me strong and gave me the courage to speak up for her even when professionals had given up on her. By sharing her journey with you I wish to carry on her teachings of unconditional love toward all who had the privilege of being in her presence. To tell you a little about our family, Trina was the little sister of Jackie and Jonathon and the youngest of my three children. Trina also had Uncle Dean and cousin Megan, whom she loved very much. When Trina was three years old I became a foster parent; after 25 years I am still a foster parent; I truly believe that because Trina couldn't be in the outside world, God brought the world to her. She will live in the hearts of all the children who came to our home.

Even though it may seem like Trina's life was only about challenges and hurdles, I hope that you feel the true meaning of the strength and endurance that she had and the miracle of her life. Everyone in this world deserves the best treatment from all of the systems that are designed to help us to be healthy and enjoy all that life has to offer.

The Bond Of Love

A baby girl was born on August 23, 1984 in a little town in Saskatchewan. One month early (actually two weeks), this tiny girl was scheduled to come into this world by C-section. (Her older sister and brother had been born the same way.) Jackie and Jonathon were so excited to have a new baby in the family. The crib was all set up for her in my bedroom.

It was extremely hot on August 20, 1984 when I went into early labour. All day I'd had so much energy—a sign that things were changing with my body. Once at the hospital, the doctors decided to try and stop the labour as the baby was still very small. Every effort was made to hold off the delivery, but this little one was coming no matter what. Two days of labour was all I could take. An amniocentesis determined that the baby's lungs were developed, so the C-section was scheduled.

I was given the choice to be awake or sleeping during the birth. Since I had been asleep for the first two children I wanted to stay awake and hold this baby as soon as he or she was born. Prepped and ready to go, I felt fear, and at the same time, excitement.

There are lots of people in the room including the baby's father. The doctors said, "Okay. Here we go. Your baby will be in your arms in a few minutes." I couldn't feel or see anything, just the pressure of the surgical knife cutting and the release of the fluid that had been protecting my little one for all these months. There was a rush of movement in the room. The doctor who delivered the baby yelled, "Oh my God, Niagara falls!" There was triple the normal amount of fluid. Nurses are threw blankets on the floor so nobody would slip and fall.

It's a girl! But she did not take her first breath and cry. All I heard was that the baby was not breathing and the rush of everyone around me. What was only a short period of time seemed like forever. Finally the baby started to cry and both baby and I could breathe. She is put in an incubator. She is so beautiful, with a full head of pure blonde hair—so tiny, but the most gorgeous baby ever. I was so eager to hold her as soon as she came into the world.

The incubator was rolled over close to my head so I could see my precious baby girl. I was given only a minute to touch her head before she was taken to the neonatal unit for babies who were not able to sustain themselves.

"This can't be happening!" I thought. I started to cry and freak out. I wanted to know what was wrong with my baby. The doctors assured me that she would be fine and that they had suctioned the fluid out of her lungs so she could breathe on her own. They told me, "We're going to put you to sleep now. We need to stitch you up."

I was crying very hard by then but was soon put under. Twelve hours later I woke up, drowsy from the morphine the doctors had given me. I wanted to get up and go see my baby. The nurses told her I could go as soon as I was able to sit up and get into a wheel chair.

I gathered the strength and will power to go to the neonatal unit to see my baby. I sat in the wheel chair and waited for the nurse to take me there. The nurse sat down on the chair

Denise F. Loewen

beside me. She says she wanted to prepare me for what she was going to see when I went down to the unit.

"The baby is going to have many tubes coming out of her little body—one in her nose to feed her, another one coming out of her mouth to drain leftover fluid from her lungs, and an intravenous drip in her head," the nurse explained. She told me what each one was doing to help keep my baby alive. I listened, but didn't really hear what the nurse was saying. All I could think was, "Let's go already! I'm fine! I just want to see my baby," although I didn't say this out loud. My head was spinning from the morphine. I was worried that the nurse might change her mind and not take me to see my baby.

Finally, it was time to go. I was sweating, nauseated, and shaking. The nurse took me down the elevator to the room that the baby was in. Once in the room, I saw lots of babies in incubators. I was taken over to the one that held my beautiful little girl. I started to cry and wanted to hold her so badly, but I was not yet allowed. I could only put my hand through the hole on the side of the incubator and touch my baby. It was very warm in the room. From the morphine and crying I felt like I was going to vomit. The nurse said that it was normal to feel that way after having surgery.

The nurse told me that it was time to go back upstairs and get some rest. I didn't want to leave, but I also felt very ill. I was taken back to my room. Getting back in the bed was not easy as the pain was overwhelming. The nurse gave me something to ease the pain from the surgery, but nothing can ease the pain of seeing my baby looking so small and weak.

I slept until the following morning. The ill feeling of the day before had all but gone. I opened my eyes and looked around at the other moms in the room. Some of them had their babies with them and looked so happy holding their little ones in their arms. At once a feeling of anxiety came over me and I wanted to go to my baby right then. I rang the bell and waited for a nurse to come. It felt like a lifetime. The C-section made it impossible for me to get out of bed on my own and to get the baby. I was told I needed to eat first and then someone would come to take her to the nursery. It didn't seem right to me because I knew how to get there, but I was told I had to be taken by a nurse. While I patiently waited for someone to come, the baby's doctor came to see me and explained what was had been happening. He assured me that the little one would be fine, but that there had been so much extra fluid around the baby that her lungs had filled up with fluid. He also said he was pleased with the birth weight of 5 lbs. 2 oz. They had originally thought the baby was going to be much smaller than she was. This was good news. He didn't say much more since, but I was having a hard time focusing on the doctor. I just wanted to know when I could be taken to see my baby.

A lady came into my room to talk to me about how scary it was to see your baby in the neonatal unit. She went on to tell me that she also understood that it was hard to be with your little one when she has tubes in them to keep her alive. She said that sometimes moms are so scared they don't want to be with their babies. I told her I was fine. I wanted to go, but nobody was coming to take me. That was the scary part, knowing that I had to wait until someone else could take me to go see my baby. The nurse assured me that someone would be there shortly and she handed me a letter. She told me it is a letter from my littlegir to me. She wanted me to read it. I told her I would but I right then I wanted to see my baby. I told her, "I need to go see her, please! Get someone to take me now."

Denise F. Loewen

Even though I had been down to see her the day before, it all seemed like a bad dream. The closer we got to the room that my baby was in, the more scared I got. I really didn't know what to expect. The tears rolled down my face before I even saw my baby girl. She was so small and the tubes looked so big on her tiny body. They had shaved all of her blonde hair off so they could put the intravenous tube into her little head. I was scared to touch her for fear that I would hurt her. The nurses knew how I was feeling and showed me that the baby would not get hurt. She needed to be touched and talked to.

That day was spent with my baby girl. I didn't even want to take the time to eat, but the nurses told me they would take very good care of my precious baby. By that evening I could get in and out of bed and wheel myself down to the neonatal unit on my own. It is amazing how one can overcome pain for the love of a child.

When I had a few minutes to myself I read the letter that was given to me by the nurse. I cried for a long time. It was hard to believe that my love could grow even stronger than it already was. The letter put the love that I already had for my new baby girl to a dimension that no one could ever understand.

A lot of other moms that came and went while I was waiting for her to get out of the neonatal unit. One of them has stayed in my heart—a mom who wanted a baby girl so badly that she only brought pink outfits and blankets to the hospital. She had already had a baby boy and was sure this one was going to be a girl, but she had given birth to a little boy. She was so upset that she couldn't stop crying. When she asked about my baby and I told her a little of what was wrong and that I just wanted her to be okay. She didn't even know what to say and went back to her room.

I spent most of my time with my baby girl. My two older children got to come to the hospital to see her, but they weren't allowed to see their new baby sister. It was so sad—they were so excited, but they also missed their mom very much. There were so many tears—I wanted to go home and be with them at home but at the same time I didn't want to miss a minute with my new baby. It just didn't seem fair.

On the third day, the tube that was draining the baby's lungs came out and this meant that the feeding tube could also come out. I was able to nurse her for the first time. We had to stay in the neonatal unit, but holding her without tubes and knowing that she was going to be okay was the best feeling in the world.

When I went back up to my room to clean up and walk around a bit, the mom with the baby boy appeared. She came into my room and handed me the cutest little pink socks. She gave me a hug and said, with tears in her eyes, that she hoped my baby would be okay and she wanted to apologize for getting so upset about having a boy instead of a girl. She went on to say she was thankful that her little boy is healthy and that she would never take that for granted. It was a beautiful moment that I will never forget. I took the little pink socks with me when I went back to hold my little one and put them on her tiny feet. I smiled while holding my little girl. She was already so loved by many people and there was no way she would not be okay.

The next morning the doctor came into my room and told me I could go home with my little one. The first emotion I had was total excitement—I missed my other two little ones so much. The doctor said that, because the baby was eating

8   *Denise F. Loewen*

fine and breathing well on her own, there was no need to stay in the hospital any longer. I thanked him and sat on my bed, not knowing what to do first. I was still in a lot of pain from the surgery, but I started to gather up my things and phoned the baby's father to tell him that they can go home. I knew that it would take him a few hours to get there so I had time to get ready.

One of the nurses brought the baby up to my room; it was so overwhelming to have my baby girl with me like all the other moms. The new friends she has made all come to see "the little peanut." This name stuck with her—she was so tiny—tiny like a peanut.

Being with my baby without all the nurses around to help with everything was very scary at first. While holding my little one and talking to her about going home to see her brother and sister, I noticed that she was starting to turn a little blue. Frightened, I buzzed for help. No one came right away and a state of panic set in. I called for someone to help and, finally, after what seemed like forever, a nurse came and looked at the baby. She told me the baby was losing her body heat needed to go back in the incubator to warm her back up. It worked. After a few minutes her colour returned to normal and I was relieved.

The nurse came back to check on us and she explained why the baby must be feed every three hours. Due to the fact that she was a premature baby and small she needed the nutrition. Nursing was going well; the baby was latching on and all seemed fine, although she took a long time to eat and it was hard to keep her awake.

Once the nurse left and I had time to think a little, some panic set in. I looked at the baby, nice and warm in the incubator, and got worried about how I was supposed to keep her warm once we got home. Again I buzzed the nurse, feeling I needed an immediate answer. The nurse came and said the baby's doctor will be there to see us before we are released. I thought, "Thank God it's summer and hot out. That should help."

When the doctor came to check the baby one more time before we were to leave, I talked to him about how to take care of her at home if she needs to be in an incubator to stay warm. The doctor told me to hold her and that my body heat would keep her warm. It made sense but I did not realize what it really meant. The doctor also made a comment that they needed the incubator in a couple of hours for another baby who was being flown in from another town and that my baby was the healthiest and biggest baby in the unit. I was confident that all would be fine. Life had never been easy, and I had overcome adversity before in my life.

Thus began my first days with my baby girl. When I started to write this life journey of my Trina I thought it would be better if I wrote it as a story instead of an account of our lives. As I wrote, I realized I couldn't do it that way. This is the life of my daughter and her journey on this Earth. I truly hope her story will reach many others and help you get through some of the toughest times in your life. Courage, strength, and harmony with your loved one are what I hope everyone will take from this very special journey.

We drove home with our new baby girl, Trina. I was so excited and scared at the same time. The weather is warm. Getting home and seeing Jackie and Jonathon is all I can think about. To me they were the most wonderful kids in the whole world. Once home, the kids were overwhelmed by their new little sister. I sat with them and let them hold her. She is so tiny. At five and two, they are babies themselves.

The rest of the day is spent holding all three of my children and trying to feed the new baby. Days go by and things were going well, but Trina did not wake up or cry. She just slept.

It was hard to keep up with all three children while nursing on a three-hour feeding schedule and the surgery was also taking a toil. There never seemed to be any time to rest. Being a young, healthy mom was a bonus and there were also other family members around. My dad and brother lived in the same little town and they would come over and help out with Jackie and Jonathon or hold Trina so I could make meals and clean or just spend some one-on-one time with the other kids. They loved their grandpa and uncle so much. Friends would come by for coffee and listen to my worries about the baby never waking up or crying.

If Trina was put down it could only be for short periods of time. She needed to be held to keep her body temperature where it should be. My grandmother, the kid's great-grandma, tried all she could to help—she made a feather quilt for the baby's bed and it helped a little bit, but I didn't feel comfortable leaving her for more than a few minutes at a time. Having Trina in a pouch on my body was the best place for her. Having her very close made me feel better.

For the first few weeks, life was all about my three children. There was no time to think about anything else. Even though things were hard, my kids were my life and never did I feel unlucky that this is what every day was like. As far as I can remember, the trips to the doctor for checkups for Trina and myself went well. The doctor was a little concerned that she wasn't really gaining weight, but he explained that, being premature, it would take a bit longer for her little body to catch up. He seemed more worried about me—he felt I needed to get more rest. I told him I was fine and assured him that I did have some help.

While my dad was not afraid to hold Trina and be left alone with her, some of my friends, and even her dad, felt uncomfortable because she was so small. I understood for the most part. There were things that scared me a little also, such as having to keep her body as upright as I could or she would make snorkel sounds as though she wasn't getting enough air. This scared me. Trina would do this at times when she was laying down flat; it was easiest to sleep with her on my chest, sitting up in a chair. As time went on it seemed to get worse; I didn't get a lot of sleep, and every breath she took would wake me up. I would listen to her all night long. It seemed that I was nursing all the time. It was hard to keep her awake and sucking. Trina hated it when I wiped her down with a damp cloth, but it would make her suck again. I was starting to get worn out—I never admitted that to anyone—being strong and taking care of my own was what I was famous for. I also worried about how much rest Trina was actually getting. My other little ones would sleep through the night and have three- to four-hour naps during the day. Because I had to wake her to feed her so frequently, Trina didn't get this undisturbed rest.

Bathing Trina was a long process. Her little body had to be done in stages, one little body part at a time. In between she had to be cuddled and warmed up. She was so beautiful and never fussed, but that was the biggest worry. Some people would say how lucky I was that she was not a crier. I didn't feel lucky—I would have rather had her crying and making a fuss. At three months old she hadn't gained any weight, which meant she was not getting stronger.

Denise F. Loewen

At her doctor's appointments I always voiced my concerns; during one appointment he asked me to stay and feed her. He wanted to make sure that she was getting milk. They weighed her before I fed her and then again after. She was eating about two ounces, which was fine for her size. What the doctor witnessed was the trouble she had breathing while nursing. He really didn't understand before what was making me so worried about this until he heard her. He then made an appointment with a specialist for her. He told me there could be something going on that needs to be looked at.

A week later, after I had fallen asleep in my bed with Trina next to me, I woke up and couldn't move. The pain in my body was so intense I felt like everything was broken. I couldn't speak; it was like I was in a coma. I could hear, but not respond. The kids were outside with their dad—I could hear them playing. I tried to yell but nothing came out. I could feel the tears running down my face. I didn't know where Trina was and she needed to be fed. I don't know how long it was that I lay there, but I heard my dad come in the house and call my name. He came into the bedroom and found me. I remember him trying to wake me up. When he shook me the pain that raced through my body was unbearable. He yelled for my husband to come in saying something was wrong and he needed to take me to the hospital.

The next thing I remember was waking up in the hospital. A nurse came into my room and told me I had been sleeping for four days. I just wanted to know where Trina was and if she was okay. I remembered I needed to feed her and couldn't move. They reassured me she was fine; they had kept her in the nurses' station so someone would be with her at all times. One nurse said that when they brought me in they thought the baby was sick also. They had been feeding her with a bottle because they couldn't wake me. When our family doctor came to see me he explained that at first they thought I had gotten an infection in my incision from the C-section. I had an extremely high fever and did not respond to anything. The tests showed no infection of any kind. What had happen was I had had a body collapse from lack of sleep. I was still sore, like someone had beaten every inch of my body. I was also very weak. They brought me my baby but I wasn't allowed to hold her unless a nurse was with me. They asked me about her and how we were doing. I tried to explain all the worries I had. A mother knows when something is not right with their child. Even though the doctors kept telling me it was because she was premature, it just seemed to be more than that.

Being young and thinking that all doctors knew everything, when they explained their ideas or thoughts to me, I just assumed they were right. Our doctor was a wonderful man; he always listened to me and never made me feel like I didn't know what I was talking about. He just didn't know what was wrong and had made a specialist appointment earlier about her eating. After this episode, he wanted a rush put on it. After a few more days in the hospital we went home. Now that Trina was being bottle fed it was easier for her to drink. We bought premature nipples so sucking would be easier for her. The doctor also recommended that she start using a soother to strengthen her jaw muscles. She didn't like it; I had to hold it in her mouth and try to keep her awake for a few minutes at a time. Her sister and brother loved to help with this task. They never wanted to leave her side. They were on a mission to make her smile and open her eyes.

Now that Trina was drinking more at a time, she started vomiting. This at first was not a big concern because that's

Denise F. Loewen

what babies do. Being bottle fed should have given me a bit more free time with Trina's dad also being able to be a part of the feedings. This didn't work out so well, however. He was afraid of her because she was so little and he didn't want to feed her. It bothered me at first, but I soon got over this issue. I didn't have the time or the energy to worry about something that I couldn't change anyway. The vomiting seemed to get worse. Every time she ate she would throw up everything. Once again we were back to the doctor's for advice. Our family doctor told me not to worry too much. He said I should feed her small amounts, but often. She seemed to be doing a little better; she had gained a few ounces. But it was still not enough—she was almost three months old and had not even gained a pound.

Going to the specialist, was scary. I wanted everything to be fine. He checked her weight and was concerned; when he heard the way she was breathing when I fed her, he was more concerned about her jaw. He examined her and said she had a condition called Pierre Robin syndrome. This was a problem that would require surgery when she was older; nothing could be done as a baby. He explained to me that her jawbones were not fully developed and that's why she had trouble breathing when laying down flat. I told him that I had stopped nursing and had her sitting up as high as I could. It was her vomiting that I was most concerned about. I also told him that she never cried or woke up for feedings. His explanation for this was that because she was so small and it was so much work for her to eat—that was all the energy she had. It didn't seem to be an issue with him. When I told him she vomited a lot, he said it looks like more than it really is. We went home thinking she would be fine.

Trina wasn't fine. The vomiting got worse. It was so bad that every couple days we were back at the hospital. She was vomiting so much that she was continuously getting dehydrated. A lot of foamy substance was coming out with the milk that she vomited. The doctors could not explain why. Oh my God—we made so many trips to the doctor. Jackie and Jonathon didn't understand why their little sister was always gone. It was so often that the first the first thing they would do when they woke up was check to see if I was home. They knew that I was always holding her and if I wasn't home their baby sister was in the hospital again.

I was so torn between being at the hospital with my baby girl or being at home with my other two wonderful children. They needed me, too. We spent every moment together that we could. Sometimes I would drive 20 minutes home from the hospital in between feedings just to sit with them and read them stories. The nurses were so nice, and they got to know all of us well. They loved all my children; even our doctor became very connected with my family. I was always anxious about leaving Trina at the hospital alone, but the nurses would keep her in the nurses' station when I had to go home to see my other children.

The same care would happen every time we were at the hospital. They would give her intravenous to get her hydrated and send her home. When we were sent to the city hospitals it was worse. The doctors in the big hospitals were not nice at all. I would explain to them about the vomiting and the foam that she would vomit out. They would suction out her lungs and sometimes tube-feed her. They never had an explanation for me as to why they suctioned out her lungs. I never wanted to leave her alone in the city hospitals. There she was in a big crib and in a room away from the nurses. Her breathing made

Denise F. Loewen

me anxious. At the city hospitals she was put on a monitor that would alarm if she stopped breathing or was choking from vomiting. The doctors treated me terribly. One doctor told me that there was nothing wrong with my baby and it seemed to him that I didn't really want her or I wouldn't bring her to the hospital all the time. I couldn't believe this. I never left her when we were there, although there was one time I did go out to eat—no one had brought me anything to eat all day. I let the nurses know that I was going out for a bit. I was gone for two hours and when I got back my baby girl had vomited and was lying in it. It had been so long that her little face was stuck to the blanket. It had dried and no one had checked on her. I was sick to my stomach. When the doctor came in to see us and told me I didn't want my baby, I got her packed up and took her home. It was then that I started to lose respect for the big city doctors.

Another time with another doctor I was told that I was probably burping her to hard and his answer was that I shouldn't hold her when I feed her and to not pick her up to burp her. This was the most ridiculous thing I had ever heard. When I told him he was wrong he didn't like this at all. I asked him if I could get one of the monitors for her at home so when I put her down I didn't have to worry so much. He looked at me and said, "Your baby needs you before she stops breathing, not after she's dead." I just stood there. I didn't even know how to respond.

Our family doctor never treated me that way; he always listened and tried to help me. He said to me one day, "We will figure it out. Just don't give up." He was so wonderful— one time when she was in the hospital he wanted me to go and see my other children. I had been crying and when he came into Trina's room he promised me he would stay with her all night so I could get a night's sleep and spend some time with my two at home. That was the nicest thing ever done for me. And he did stay all night with her like he said he would. I felt like I could continue fighting for her. He told me he understood more about her breathing and I didn't have to constantly explain it to him.

She never cried and very seldom opened her eyes. Thinking about all this now, I can't believe no one but me realized how sick she was. Looking at her you could tell she was not well. She was so tiny; she had only gained a pound in over three months. It all seems like a bad nightmare now. Being scared for my baby everyday was so mentally draining.

I had a friend who was a nurse and she would listen to me and go through her medical books trying to find something that fit. One day she called me and said she thought she had found something that seemed like it could be the problem that Trina had. I was so excited; finally I had something that I could take to the doctors. We had an appointment with a pediatrician in a few days. I could only hope that we would be home long enough to make the appointment. I would be sick to my stomach most of the time when we had specialist appointments. It seemed that they thought I was crazy and an over protective mother and I needed to stop worrying about every little thing. I just couldn't accept that it was all because she was premature. To me it was more than that.

We made it to the pediatrician's appointment. He looked at her weighed her and said he thought she was fine, even though she had not gained any weight. I remember being so nervous. I wanted to shout out what was wrong with her, but I had to be careful. He had been cruel to me before. I helped him in the examining room, patiently keeping my mouth shut and waiting for him to finish. Finally, I asked him if he could

Denise F. Loewen

check to see if she had pyloric stenosis. I explained to him that my friend was a nurse and she agreed with me that it could be why Trina was vomiting all the time. I'll never forget his response—he leaned close to me and looked right at me and said, "There is no way she could have that because it only happens to boys." He said it so matter-of-factly, I didn't know how to respond. I was sick inside. I really thought we had figured it out. I just went home once again with my little girl. It took an hour to get home from the city and I always worried about her while I was driving. It was a long time for her not to be in my arms. I didn't know what to think. I remember wanting to scream and cry. We were in and out of the hospital so often that I lost count. I was scared most of the time, scared to put her down, scared to fall asleep. I was torn between my two little ones at home and my baby in the hospital. I knew the older children missed me and I tried to give them 200 per cent when I was at home, or even when they were at the hospital with me. The only time I would leave her even for a little while was when she was in the hospital where our family doctor was. He seemed to be the only one who agreed with me. He would keep her in his hospital if he could get her stable, and if he couldn't off we would go to the city. We saw so many different doctors it seems like a blur to me at times.

I know it sounds like I was a single parent, but I wasn't. The kid's dad was not really available for the baby. He never felt comfortable with her. He did spend as much time as he could with the other two children. For that I am grateful. I also had a great dad and brother whom my children loved. When they couldn't watch the kids, my friends were always there for us. Trina's first Christmas came and went. When we went to get pictures taken with Santa, he didn't want to hold her—he said she was too small for him. I just smiled and said that was okay. I held her and stood beside him. She was four months old and I realized then how tiny she was. I was just used to her being small and I didn't notice how intimidating her size was for other people. She was still like a newborn baby.

Still nothing had changed. We would be at home for a few days and back at the hospital for a few. This became our lives; I learned to do everything with her in a pouch. I felt like a mother kangaroo. She always had to be bundled up warm and close to my body. Thank God for family and friends. I tried to take better care of myself. The last thing I ever wanted to experience again was a collapse. It was so painful and frightening. It wasn't just me being that sick, but mostly it was the first time I was not able to take care of my kids. That was the scariest feeling.

Putting this into words is very difficult. I guess while living this I never really thought about how hard it was to get through each day. We just did it, and for that again I'm grateful.

Even with the way things were, we also had a lot of fun. The kids loved to dance and sing and would sing to their baby sister. When she would stay awake and smile at them, they would laugh and hug her. They were so small themselves— amazing children, that's what they were. No doubt about it. We would sit together and read stories for hours. I'll never forget how lucky I felt. I suppose I really didn't realize just how sick my baby was. This was, I think, a blessing; I would have felt unable to care for her the way I was If I knew. I do remember thinking after talking with the doctor that said he didn't think I wanted her, "Could they take her away from me?" I believe that gave me an inner strength to do whatever

Denise F. Loewen

I had to do keep my baby safe from them. What a horrible way to feel. I now I tried to keep her home more. I would always confide in our family doctor and beg him not to send her back to the same pediatricians. He was so great. He'd say, "Don't worry. We will figure it out." I think if it hadn't been for him she would not have lived to see her first birthday— actually I know that for a fact. There was so much more going on in our lives, it doesn't seem possible to have lived it all. That is for another time I guess, if I ever have it in me to share that part of my life.

I could tell that Trina was getting sicker. As a mom you just know these things. Back at the hospital once again, our family doctor made some calls to other pediatricians. He was consulting with them asking them for advice. He came back to us at the hospital and told me there was a pediatrician who had agreed to see her. She was six months old now and still did not cry. She was not even strong enough to hold her head up by herself. The doctor said he would see her but we had to go to the city right away. She was stable enough to make the drive. I don't remember if I went by myself or if her dad came with me. I had hope once again. Now it seems crazy to think that every time we saw a new doctor I would have hope once again. I did watch what I said, though—that I remember.

When we got to his office I recognized him. He was the pediatrician who took care of my first baby Jackie when she was born. He was a nice man. I was a single young mom and I remember him talking to me and explaining everything that had gone wrong with the birth of my first. He didn't make me feel less than because I was single. I remember feeling that I could be the best mom ever. I didn't think he remembered me and I didn't ask him. I just wanted him to focus on Trina with no distractions. He asked me to put her on the table and get her undressed. I looked at him and told him I couldn't take all her clothes off at the same time. She would get to cold. I wasn't sure how he was going to respond; I kind of held my breath. I really needed him to see what I saw and not think I was just an over-protective mom. He looked at me and said, "That's fine—we can do it slowly." He examined her head to toe. He measured her body and her head. When he was done—oh my God I can hardly breathe now just thinking about it—he sat down and told me my baby had what he called failure to thrive. I didn't quit understand and stayed silent. All I could do was shake my head to let him know I was listening. He said she was starving to death. I almost fainted. I held her so tight. He went on to say he was going to hospitalize her immediately. He was going to give himself 24 hours to figure out what the problem was. If he couldn't in that amount of time, he was going to transfer her to the children's hospital in Toronto.

I was shaking hard, I knew she was sick, but even I didn't know how sick she really was. He told me she didn't cry or even stay awake because her little body was too weak. He also told me she was doing as well as she was because I was still feeding her with bottles for premature babies. This made it easier for her to suck, even though she was throwing it back up; she was actually living on the milk that stuck to the lining of her stomach. I asked him about the foam that she vomited up. He said he did not know why, but he was going to figure it out. From his clinic we went straight to the hospital. Things were so different with him. He phoned the hospital and told them we were coming. Everyone was so nice to me. It seemed unreal. I was so grateful. A few hours after being at the hospital, a nurse came in our room and explained that she was going to take my tiny little one for some tests. I couldn't come with her but I would have time to get something to eat. I forgot to eat most of the time. I never wanted to leave her. Sometimes the nurses would bring me food and sometimes not. It all depended if they thought I was crazy or not. I really didn't care what they thought most of the time. I got a coffee and hurried back to her room. It seemed like forever, but they finally brought her back. The nurse told me her doctor would be in to talk to me. I was so scared, wondering if he didn't find out what was wrong if she would be able to last. I took her out of the crib. She really looked so small in there. At home she was in a baby's bassinet.

There was another baby who had come into the hospital room while I was out. When they brought Trina back, the other mom said, "Oh my gosh! Did you just have her?" When I told her she was six months old she couldn't believe it. Her baby was three months old and was huge compared to Trina. We talked a little bit; I told her how hard it was to get a doctor to believe me. She gave me a hug and said it would be okay. I just smiled and said I hoped so.

The doctor came in a little while later; I'm not even sure how long it was. He came in and smiled at me. He said they had found the problem and they would be able to fix it. He also said he was sorry, but she would have to have surgery. By this time it was getting late. He told me they would operate first thing in the morning. I remember him touching her head and saying she was going to be just fine. I asked what the surgery was for and I'll never forget what went through my body when he said she had pyloric stenosis. I looked at him and I said I thought that only happen to boys. He replied it is normally a boy's decease but they have found it in girls. It was very rare, but it could happen. He smiled and said,

"Don't worry," and touched my shoulder. I couldn't wait for the morning, but I was also very scared.

Morning came, but I hadn't slept. I held Trina and rocked her in the rocking chair all night. When they came to get her they explained what would be done and where the incision would be. They said she would be in surgery for about half an hour or so. They were taking extra precautions because she was so small. I waited and waited. I called home to let my family know that she was in surgery. I was hungry but couldn't make myself leave the floor. It seemed like she was gone a lot longer than they said she would be. I walked around that room so many times, I'm sure I wore a hole in the floor.

Finally they came into the room, wheeling her crib in. I saw her and started to cry, she was so small. They had her hands tied to the crib, there was intravenous in her head. It was put there because her veins were too small. I didn't know what to do. I couldn't hold her. I asked why her hands were tied. The nurse smiled and said, "She's a feisty little one. She didn't like the tubes and was trying to pull them out." They looked at me and said, "You have a real little fighter there." Later—I don't know how much later, as time seemed like a blur—her doctor came in to see her.

He explained that the surgery took longer than they expected. The reason why was because the surgeons hands were too big to fit into the incision that would normally have been made. They had to cut her right down to her belly button and this took a little bit longer. Because she was so small they could only give her a certain amount of anesthetic. Everything had taken longer than planned. He looked at me and said, "She has one strong heart. She woke up before they had finished stitching her up and they couldn't give her any more anesthetic because of her size." He was very proud of her for doing so well. He assured me she was going to be just fine. The valve that went from her esophagus to her stomach was actually missing. They had to cut the stomach muscle and wrap it around her esophagus. This way when she ate and her stomach contracted to digest her food, the muscle that was wrapped around the esophagus would shut the tube and the food couldn't come back up. He also said they put in a plastic valve that would work while her body healed; as she grew the plastic valve would not work but it wouldn't bother anything. The muscle would take over the job. He kept saying he couldn't believe how strong her heart was and if it hadn't been she might not have made it through the surgery. He said he wanted us to stay for a few days, but from how she was doing he felt there would not be any further problems. I looked at her and knew she would be fine.

We stayed at the hospital, and then the tubes finally came out. She started eating on her own and did not vomit. I was so happy that she was going to live, that's all I could think about. She was eating and not vomiting! Nothing could take that happiness from me. I remember telling them I understood and would make sure to have her checked often. I knew I would anyway. I just couldn't stop smiling. I really don't even remember going home; I know that sounds crazy, but my next memory is just being at home sitting with my three babies on the couch.

The next trip to the doctor would be to take out the stitches. And to weigh her and see how much weight she gained and not how much she didn't. It was a true miracle. The next visit to see her pediatrician was amazing. My baby had already started to gain weight. She had not vomited again. I couldn't stop thanking him. I told him he was my first baby's doctor, I knew he didn't remember and that was fine with me. He was very proud and happy for us. He was wonderful—he took the time to explain everything to me all over again. He also told me to remember that it would take longer for her outer body to show weight gain. Her inner body had to catch up and heal first. He also said this is like a new birthday for her. Even though she was six months old, she hadn't had a chance to develop the way she should have. I did get the nerve to tell him I had asked another doctor if it could be pyloric stenosis and he wouldn't even check because of the boy thing. I said she was three months then. He didn't really say anything but said that it was a good thing I didn't quit trying to get help for her. I guess doctors stick together. I didn't want him to do anything; I just wanted him to know a little bit about how we were treated. I thanked him for everything he did for us. He wanted to see her again in a month. I would take my little miracle baby home and start living our life the way it should have been right from the day she was born.

Never did a baby get as many hugs and kisses as she did. She grew every day. Every day she got stronger and became more alert. She started smiling and staying awake. Yeah, even crying. It was the most wonderful sound I had ever heard.

My baby girl was supposed to live. I didn't know it then but she was going to change a lot of lives. All I knew was that I was right and they were wrong. I knew I should never give up. We as moms and dads know our children. We have built-in radar and we need to trust ourselves. If I had listened to all those doctors who said there was nothing wrong with her and it was all in my head Trina would probably have been gone about two weeks from the day of her surgery.

For the next few months I took her to see the doctor who saved her life. Every time we went Trina's weight had gone

Denise F. Loewen

up, she was more alert, and was doing well. One of her examinations was exceptionally great. Her doctor took extra time with her. He got her to smile; he checked her toes and fingers. He told me to watch something. He put a pencil under her little toes and she curled them around the pencil. I just looked at him not quite knowing what he was showing me. He looked at me and said, "See how her toes curl around the pencil?" I said, "Yes," He said, "Don't ever let anyone tell you she isn't smart." I just smiled and said, "Okay." I didn't know then how important that one comment was going to be to my baby and me. That comment stayed in my heart forever.

Faith Is The Knowledge Within The Heart, Beyond The Reach Of Proof

It was so amazing being at home every day with my kids. They were all growing happy and now healthy. There was no more throwing up; now that she had gained weight and strength, Trina could now hold her own body heat. She was such a happy baby, smiling all the time.

I still had a hard time putting her down. It was like she was part of me; I had her attached to me for so long that I felt there was something missing when I wasn't carrying her. It was much easier caring for the kids. Jackie sister would sit on the couch and hold Trina like she never wanted to let her go. Jonathon, although still a baby himself, was so gentle with her it made me want to cry with pride. So many people told me when Trina was in and out of the hospital and I had to leave the older two so much that they were going to resent her and not bond with her. They told me the kids would be angry and they would feel Trina took me away from them. Never did I see any resentment from them. They were eager to help with anything for her. They would even sit with her and hold her sucky in her mouth for her. We did this often throughout the day. The doctor was right when he said it would help strengthen her jaw muscles. It did help, she was able to suck better and drink a full bottle without falling asleep. She was so small when she sat in her highchair that we had to put blankets around her so she wouldn't fall over. She loved to sit and watch everything. She was always watching, smiling, and taking everything in.

At eight months old we went to see her doctor for another check up. He was very pleased with how she was doing. She was still almost 10 pounds—maybe that doesn't seem like much, but for me it was a huge. At this visit her doctor was a little concerned about her jaw and said it would be a good thing if a genetics physician were to see her. He told me he didn't think there was anything to worry about, but he would feel better checking because of her jaw development. I took her to the hospital for some blood work. My doctor said someone would call me to make an appointment when they had the results from. I'm not sure how long it took, a week maybe longer, but we did get a call. The genetics doctors wanted us to come to the city and see them. They would explain the results of her blood work then. When we went to the appointment I can't really remember thinking much about it. My little baby was doing well; she was growing and advancing. I wasn't worried about the appointment.

At the hospital and we were taken to a large room where there was a huge table with a lot of people sitting around it. I was a little nervous then—I didn't understand why so many people where there. We sat down, I'm holding Trina, and she's sleeping in my arms. Everyone thanks us for coming and they all introduced themselves. I still didn't know why we were asked to come. Finally, one of the doctors started talking about Trina's blood work and what they found was that she had a syndrome called Noonan syndrome. They explained

30   *Denise F. Loewen*

that it was hereditary and that either my husband or I had passed it on to her.

I was speechless. I don't remember saying a lot; in fact, I don't recall anything else that was said. I just remember holding Trina tighter. I recall one of the doctors getting up and sitting beside me. She looked at me and smiled at my baby and said, "I know this is a lot to understand." She offered therapy to help deal with what they had just told me about Trina. I looked at all the people watching me and I told them I was fine, I didn't need any therapy. I said that I loved her when I came into this room and I would love her even more when I left. I remember asking if she was sick and if she would have to be put in the hospital. One of the doctors said it wasn't that she was sick, but that she may not develop like other kids. I stood up and thanked them and that we would be fine. I don't know why I didn't ask any more questions; I know now I should have.

Really when I think about it today it wouldn't have made any difference to me unless she needed surgery or there was something they could fix. Driving home thinking about the name of the syndrome they said she had was odd to me. Our family doctor's name was Noonan. I don't know if I was in denial, but I never really talked about it much. The words her pediatrician said to me, "Don't ever let anyone tell you she isn't smart," played over and over in my brain.

It's strange how the mind works—it was like it never really happened. We went home and never saw those doctors again. She wasn't sick anymore so I suppose I didn't feel a need to see them. Life was great; we only had to see our family doctor after that. When I told him about the syndrome and what it was called his face revealed shock. He said he had never heard of it and that he would be there to help us with whatever we needed. That's all I needed was to know. I was at peace and nothing was going to take that away from my children or me.

By the time Trina turned one year old she was very tiny, but full of life. She was a social butterfly and won the hearts of everyone around her. Her sister and brother adored her. We were a normal family; my six-year-old daughter was in grade one. My son who was three was a wonderful little boy. They loved playing with Trina and making her laugh. Even though my little one had problems when she was born, she was growing and developing at a good pace.

She was a little slow at walking, but once she got it, away she went. It was so cute to see her walking; she was so small—about 12 to 14. I sewed, so it was easier to make her cloths myself. It was hard to find cloths to fit her nicely. She loved to do somersaults—the big game at our house. She was so loving and cuddly. I was so happy with my little family. I loved my kids so much—they were and are my life. Their dad worked with the kids' uncle on a farm away from home but was home on the weekends.

Then one morning something seemed off with the baby. When she went down for her nap she was a little warm and when she woke up she had a fever. I took her to the doctor. (Back then you could make an appointment and see your doctor that same day.) He examined her and said she had an infection in her throat. He put her on penicillin and said it was really nothing to worry about—she would be fine in a few days. We picked up her antibiotics and went home. I gave the kids lunch and put baby down for a nap and checked on her soon after. (I always checked on her while she slept—a force of habit, I guess. When your baby is born sick I don't think you really ever get over the hovering. I never thought

Denise F. Loewen

that was a bad thing.) She did not look good; her face looked swollen and her color was off. I phoned the hospital and explained to them how she was. They said it sounded like an allergic reaction to the penicillin. I took her to the hospital where they put her on IV and watched her closely. The next day she looked better so they gave me a different kind of antibiotic and we got to go home. They said to watch her closely for a few days, but that she should be fine. Jackie was also allergic to penicillin. Trina should not have been given it, but, of course, it's one of those things that happen. Thank god she was okay.

A few days later, things seemed to be fine. Her fever was gone and she was a little more chipper. She was so amazing— even when she was sick she was happy. We ate lunch, then I put her in her walker chair. When she wasn't feeling well she didn't walk as well. Her eyelids seemed to not open all the way. She had to tilt her head up a little so she could see where she was going. The doctors told me it was because she was premature as a baby. They had also told me it should correct itself as she grows; it never did. She did amazingly well, considering she had to adapt her posture to see in front of herself. If I walked too far away from her she would lift her head up and usually fall on her little bum. Her sister and brother were always there to catch her. They never really strayed far from their sister. I was sitting on the couch with her brother, reading him a story. I looked at Trina and she seemed to be staring. When I talked to her she didn't even blink. This scared me. It was like she was frozen. I panicked and rushed her to the hospital. By the time we got there she seemed fine. The doctor felt that maybe she'd had a seizure. He said by the way I described her actions, to him it seemed as though it could have been a focal seizure. He explained

Mommy, Please Don't Listen To Them　　　33

that because she'd had an infection with a fever, this could have caused her body to seizure. He also told me that most children outgrow this tendency by the time they are two to three years of age. He told me she might have them while she is fighting off the infection and to keep an eye on her. He told me that the seizures would not hurt her and should only last a minute or so. He said if she has one and it goes on for several minutes to bring her back.

That was her first seizure and I hoped it would be the last. (I didn't know anything about seizures.) I watched her all the time and didn't see her have any more. Her infection went away and once again she seemed fine. She was back to her old self, happy and full of energy. The months went by and everything was going great. Again, the kids were growing, happy, and healthy.

There was something about my Trina that was bothering me; I was worried about her vision and her jaw. Her teeth came in on time she seemed to everyone to be just fine. Christmas came and it was wonderful. The kids got everything and more. I was so grateful to have a job that I could do at home, and that I could be with my kids every day.

There were a few ear infections during the next year. I know that doesn't seem like a big deal, but for her it was. Along with the infections came fevers and then seizures. I learned as much as I could about seizures. The doctors didn't seem to be too worried. They explained that as long as they only came with a fever she would probably still outgrow them. I did everything in my power to keep her healthy and I felt that I was doing a good job. All in all, my kids were very healthy children. Trina continued to grow and started talking; it seemed like they were right about her catching up. She was potty trained at two; her speech was slow but she

Denise F. Loewen

was improving as time went on. Most of her speech was one-to three-word sentences.

Trina's doctor wanted her to see a therapist. He felt having someone see her and show me different things to do with her would help her catch up. Her therapist spent a couple hours a week with us at our home. She would watch Trina interact with the other kids and see how she communicated with them and me. Most of the things she taught me were great. I used them and felt good about it. There was one thing that bothered me. It was when her therapist told me I had to be stricter with her because she was not listening like she should be. It was very hard for me to do this. She had been through so much in her little life. She was never bad or mean or anything like that. She just didn't do things that I asked her to do all the time. By then she was only two. I felt she was such a gentle child; not listening all the time was the least of our problems.

We all communicated together, her therapist, her doctor, and myself. Health-wise things were going great. Everyone was pleased that she was gaining weight and progressing in all areas. The therapist brought up that it might be a good idea for Trina to go to daycare a few days a week. Inside, I smiled; I really knew she wanted me to do this because she thought I spoiled her and that was why she didn't listen as well as expected. However, I agreed. I would do anything if it would help. The therapist seemed to know what she was doing and I trusted her.

We found a daycare that would take her; they worked with other kids who had many different problems. Before she could start I had to get a physical done for her. This was mandatory for all kids who went to daycare. Never in my wildest dreams did I expect to find what we did during this physical.

Her doctor and I talked about the main reason why she was going to daycare as he examined her. Things went well until her looked in her ears. We talked about the ear infections that she'd had over the last year. He said her ears were almost completely plugged. This was due to the infections causing her ears not to drain properly. He did a simple hearing test on her. He asked her where's mommy. He said this to her when she wasn't looking at him. She didn't respond, and then he got her to look at his face and asked her again. She pointed to me. He just smiled and said what a smart little girl I had. She was reading lips and that was why she didn't always listen. He couldn't believe how well she could sing her nursery rhymes, but could not speak a full sentence. I think it was because whatever I tried to teach her I did with music. She loved it and responded to it. It made sense; in doing therapy with her, one of the things I was told to do was to make eye contact with her when asking her to do things. The doctor laughed he said she sure fooled everyone. Even her therapist didn't pick up on it and she was trained to watch for things like that. Her doctor said she would need tubes put in her ears, this would keep the wax from building up and then she should be able to hear fine. He wanted me to take her to an eye, ear, and throat specialist for some tests and to arrange for the surgery.

When we went for that appointment the specialist said she had no hearing in her left ear and only about 40 percent in her right. She had the tubes put in a few weeks later. The surgery went well and the doctor was pleased. He said the tubes would stay in her ears for about a year and then would fall out. It was important to have her ears checked often to see if she would need to have more put in—this was normal and I was told not to worry if she needs them put in again.

Denise F. Loewen

We also talked a little about her eyes and how they didn't open all the way. He explained it was because her eyelids didn't have folds. There was a fairly simple surgery that could fix this condition, but he also said she was too young—the youngest child who'd had the surgery had been five years old. We talked about how it was affecting her walking and her fear of losing me when I stood too far from her. We set up another appointment to talk about it further.

It was amazing—when got home she was a different kid. She no longer turned the stereo and TV up all the time. When I called her even from another room she would come. How wonderful this was, and also a relief because she was such a great kid and I didn't have to feel guilty about the disciplining strategies I was told to do. I never felt comfortable with it and it felt good that I was right. She didn't need to be disciplined for not listening. It was all good. Her talking became clearer and although she still didn't talk in complete sentences, I was sure that would come in time. It's funny how life happens. If her therapist hadn't suggested daycare, who knows how long Trina would have been nearly deaf and how would she have been treated as though she was not listening? I don't even like to think about the what-ifs. I did start to realize how important it is to listen to others, not always give my opinion, even if I thought I was right. Things could have been turned out a lot differently if I had given attitude when I didn't agree with everything I was being told. I listened, learned, and took what I felt right for my daughter.

As it turned out she did need tubes one more time when she was around four and a half. She was in daycare when I started to notice she was being disciplined for not listening. I knew right away what the problem was. I took her to the doctor and sure enough she needed tubes again. I grew a little more with this experience. I learned just how important it was to always be present in some ways when others are taking care of your child. I would go and observe her at her daycare to see how she was doing. When I saw what was happening with my own eyes it was very clear. If I hadn't seen it myself it may have continued without my knowledge.

We went to the specialist about her having the eye surgery. He didn't want to do it until she was bigger. He said the cartilage they would use to place into her eye lids to hold them open and to make the fold was usually taken from the child's own legs. Trina was still very tiny for her age, but I wanted it done as soon as possible. I wanted her to have every advantage to catch up with her development as possible. He agreed to talk with another doctor about it before he would give me a decision. He was very clear that he didn't want to do it, because they would have to use cartilage from a donor.

I got a phone call from him a few weeks later and he had decided they would do it for her. He would schedule the surgery and she would need to have a physical just before the surgery—if she had any kind of illness they would postpone it. That was fine with me. Her surgery was scheduled a couple months later. After seeing the difference in her after she could hear, I was nervous and happy. I could only imagine how this was going to make her life better.

We had to be at the hospital by 7 am. The surgery was scheduled for 9:30 am. that day. The anesthesiologist came to talk to me before Trina went into surgery. He explained to me that they were going to have to give her a little bit more anesthetic than they had originally planned. This was because she had woken up during her stomach surgery. He said it would be devastating if she were to wake up during eye surgery. They would take extra precautions and he felt everything would be just fine. He showed me what they would do to open her eyelids further. They would put a small incision above her eyebrow and another one on the eyelid itself. They would be very tiny and would not be noticeable once healed. The cartilage would be placed under the skin from the eyelid and threaded up above the eyebrow. When she opened her eyes the lift of the forehead would pull the eyelids open further. He assured me this surgery had been done many times. It would not take long. Trina was given a small shot to make her sleepy and she went into the OR shortly after that. I was told to wait in the waiting room for someone to come and get me. They told me as soon as she woke up they would let me be with her.

I waited for what seemed forever—it was about an hour after they had taken her into surgery. I knew it shouldn't have been this long and I started to get a little worried—it seemed like they should have come to get me by then. I kind of got a sick feeling and started to pace. (Even now I am getting that feeling just thinking about it.) Finally, a nurse came into the waiting room. She said she was sorry no one had come to get me yet. Trina was still in recovery and they were having a hard time getting her to wake up. Normally no one is allowed in the recovery room, but they thought if she heard my voice she may respond and wake up. I was lead in to the recovery room where my little girl was on a big bed. I sat down on a chair beside her and started taking to her and saying, "Trina, it's Mommy. Come on baby it's time to wake up." I tried everything I could think of—talking, rubbing her body—I was even washing her with a cool cloth. Nothing.

I started to get scared. The nurses kept coming over and checking Trina's vital signs. Things were fine that way, but she was not responding at all. A doctor came in and checked her;

she was concerned and told me they were going to give her a shot of something. (I don't remember what it was called.) It was supposed to counteract the anesthetic and make her body wake up. They did this, we waited, and I talked to her and rubbed her little arms and hands. She did not stir. I'm sick, crying, and begging God to please help her wake up. I was blaming myself for wanting the surgery to be done. I just didn't know what to think. Doctors now were coming in often. They would check her and talk together. I just sat there holding her. Her little eyes were wide open, but she was not responding. Hours went by, they decided to give her one more shot of the medication to wake her. I think I stopped breathing. They gave her the shot and said they could not give her anymore if this didn't work. Over an hour went by. I was so scared I didn't even want to ask them what would happen if she didn't wake up soon. I just talked to her. I sang. It was like we were the only two people in the room.

Then, oh my God, I think I yelled when she moved her head. The nurses came over they were smiling and talking to her. I then realized how much trouble she was really in. I knew it had not been good, but seeing their reaction made it even more real. She woke up fast after that. She reached for my face and tried to sit up. I am thankful to this day. We were taken back to her room once she became fully awake.

Trina ate and sat in her bed. I stayed with her and cuddled her. She had the most beautiful eyes. The colour of them was an eye colour I'd never seen before. They were green with blue and brown flecks in them, and a dark blue ring around the outside. Now I could see them like never before. I never wanted to let her go again. Her nurse came in and showed me how to take care of her eyes. The cartilage was keeping her eyes from closing. She couldn't even blink. They explained

Denise F. Loewen

that for a few weeks I had to put salve in her eyes to keep them moist. Once the swelling went down from the surgery she would be able to close her eyes as normal.

It was already the end of the day. Most of it was spent in the recovery room. We had a good night and Trina slept all night with no problems. The next day when we woke up she wanted to get out of bed right away. I was a little scared to let her go and I walked behind her in case she fell. It was amazing—her balance was better already. We walked around. I stayed close but she seemed just fine. We found our way to the playroom. I sat and watched her, she was so happy pointing to everything. She was going around the room looking at things like she had never seen such things before. Even when she looked up she didn't fall down like she normally would.

Her doctor came in to see her. He was standing by the little table I was sitting at. He didn't say anything at first and I have to admit that I was terrified about what he was going to say about Trina not waking up the way she was should have. He sat down on one of the little chairs beside me and didn't say anything at first. He was just watching Trina play. He looked at me and said, "I owe you an apology." He was very pleased with how she was doing already. He didn't expect her to be up and out of bed yet, never mind in the playroom playing. That made me feel so good about my decision. I could feel her confidence growing already. Her doctor also explained that they had given her a little too much anesthetic for her size. He mentioned again how important it was that she not wake up during her surgery. I told him I was really scared, "But look at her," I said. She came over to me and sat on my lap. He talked to her for a bit, telling her how beautiful her eyes were. He smiled at me and said we could go home the next morning if her night went well. He looked at her and said, "I'm sure she'll be just fine."

We did go home the next morning. I picked up her sister and brother from my aunt and uncle's and went home. They were very excited to see her. They kept saying, "Trina can see us now, right?" They couldn't stop touching her. A few weeks later the swelling was gone and Trina was able to blink again. She started running overnight. (Well, it seemed that way.) She no longer panicked when I was too far away from her. The best thing was, she could go up and down stairs all by herself like a big girl. It was so fun for her she would just go up and down for no reason. When I think back now, she stopped turning upside down all the time. She loved to put her head on the floor and look at things upside down. I wonder if she could see more that way. It's funny how kids will adapt and find their own ways to make life better for themselves—even as an adult I had never put it together until now. She was an amazing kid who surprised me every day. I felt like the luckiest parent on Earth. Who could want more? I had three beautiful children who were loving and kind to each other and to all who came into our lives.

Denise F. Loewen

A Mother's Intuition Vs. Medical Authority

Moving to British Columbia was a big change for our family. It was scary leaving the doctors who were familiar. Things were good, though and I felt the hardest times were behind us. The children were young and would adapt. They were going to miss their grandpa so much. It was hard to leave and move so far away. My brother, the kid's uncle, and his baby girl moved with us and this made it easier. We were very close and helped each other with our kids and the ups and downs of life.

Trina was in good health. I found a daycare for her—she did very well there and the staff loved her. She was so sweet and a real social butterfly. She was developing at a rapid pace. Trina was diagnosed with being developmentally delayed. There really was no reason to think otherwise—she'd had such a rough start in life and was doing exceptionally well, considering. While attending daycare she received assessments for speech and for motor skills. Her speech came slow; she still could sing better than talk. It was recommended that we start to teach her sign language. Trina picked up on this very quickly, the only problem was she would only sign the words she could speak and would sign instead of verbalizing. This did not work out as planned so we stopped using sign language.

While there teachers from a huge school in Montreal came to our city. They were from Giant Steps, a foundation that specialized in working with autistic children. Trina's daycare was a child development center so they came to assess the children here. Trina was assessed and did not qualify for their program—they said she was not autistic and did not fit their criteria. That was fine with me; I didn't know a lot about autism. I would learn more about it as the years went on.

The next year Trina went through a few good growing spurts. She was still very small for her age, but she ate well and her body seemed to be catching up. At the age of around four Trina started to have focal seizures now and again. They were coming often enough that our new family doctor sent us to a pediatrician. We took her for an EEG to see what was going on with her brain. They couldn't find anything at the time. Still, she was definitely having seizures so her pediatrician put her on a medication for seizure activity. This medication was called Dilantin. We had her on this medication for a little over a year. She didn't seizure often, but still did. Her seizures were quick and always focal.

The time came to start getting Trina ready for kindergarten. Jackie and Jonathon went to the school by our house, so that's where I wanted Trina to go, too. Because her speech was delayed and she had seizures, she would need a one-on-one teaching assistant at school. Things went quite well at school. Trina loved it and wanted to go every day. She was so proud of her little backpack, and also loved seeing her sister and brother there.

Something changed. Things had been going so well, but I started to notice a difference in Trina's behavior. She would get frustrated easily and clench her fists and yell. There never seemed to be a reason for it—it was mostly out of the blue.

Denise F. Loewen

Because she was a calm and loving kid, this was out of the norm for her. Her eating also seemed to change. She didn't want food with any taste—all she wanted was potatoes, cornflakes, and milk. Oh my God—she couldn't get enough milk. I also noticed when she brushed her teeth her gums would bleed and her eating got worse.

Trina also needed glasses at this time; her eye specialist told us not to force her to wear them if she didn't like them at first. Well she loved them; they were the first thing she put on in the morning and the last thing she took off at night.

Trina was still having seizures even though she was on medication for this. Things began to get worse very fast. She was growing and learning, but something was just not right. The more time that passed, the more often we had to go to doctors. When we went to see her pediatrician our concern was her gums bleeding.

She started to get cavities even though she was so young (she was five years old); her front tooth had a cavity right in the front. Her dentist told us it was from the medication she was on. Talking to her doctor about this she told us he was right—that was one of the side effects from the Dilantin. The bleeding was a bad sign--it could cause her to get gum decease and lose her teeth. This was not acceptable! Since the medication was not working, her pediatrician wanted her to be seen by a neurologist at Children's Hospital. She was sure they could help us and get her on the proper medications.

When we got to Children's Hospital she was examined by the neurologist; they did an EEG on her brain to see if they could find where her seizure activity was. The tests do not show any seizure activity. The doctor does not seem to know what to do. He explained that she did not have epilepsy and that was why the medication she was on did not work. He wanted to do more tests, saying there must have been some kind of brain damage to cause the seizures. Another reason he didn't think epilepsy was she only had seizures while she was sleeping.

I wasn't sure what to think. I went over everything with him that had happened since I got pregnant with her. He even wanted to know about my other children and my pregnancies with them. I remember wanting to go home; Trina was not happy there and I was missing my other kids. The tests were done and nothing showed up. Her brain was normal.

We had another meeting with him and he told us that because brain damage was not the cause of the seizures, it had to be epilepsy. I thought this was a little strange, but I didn't know a lot about it at that time. (I also still thought doctors were the ones who knew what they were talking about and I trusted them.)

While we were at the hospital I was able to watch some videos. There were also other patients who I was able to talk to—they were outpatients who had seizures. Some of them had the same focal seizures as Trina. While talking with them, a young girl tried to explain what she felt while she was in a seizure. She said it was like being in a black space. What helped her come back to reality was when her mom would talk to her. When she heard her mom's voice, she didn't understand why, but it would get her back. I always remembered this and talked to Trina in a calm voice whenever she went into a seizure. It did seem to help, and it also made me feel better. When your child has a seizure you feel so helpless. It doesn't matter if it happens 10 times a day—every time is as hard as the first. Knowledge is what helped me feel like I had a little control, not just helping her through each seizure, but really understanding what the doctors were

Denise F. Loewen

saying, and having a conversation with them instead of just listening and nodding my head. The more information I had, the more confident I became with asking questions when I didn't understand. I no longer felt intimidated by the white coats and certificates on their walls. I was her mom and I had the best knowledge about my child.

Changes and Challenges

The doctor took Trina off the Dilantin seizure medication and put her on one called Tegretol. He said the side effects were not like those from Dilantin. He also said they had a lot of luck with other children on this medication. We talked for a while longer and he asked a lot of questions about her health at birth. When we were done I felt good about the changes. Before we left he said he would like her to be seen by the genetics team at the hospital. He wanted them to see her because of the Noonan syndrome she had been diagnosed with when she was eight months old. He told us he would set it up and they would call us for a time when we should bring Trina back. I recall thanking him and I took my little girl home. I always felt like everything was going to be just fine. We had gotten help from the best doctors. They all seemed to know what they were talking about. If only I knew then what I know now.

Trina did have to get her front tooth pulled out and also have a few fillings. The Dilantin had really destroyed her teeth and gums in a very short period of time. She had to have this done at the hospital and be put under. She just did not understand what was being asked of her at the dentist office. Even though she was five years old, she could not talk enough to express herself and didn't have to mental maturity to follow the verbal instructions. She was still much delayed in development and now was starting to show anger and frustration.

Another change that I started to notice with my gentle, loving little girl was that she didn't want to be touched as much and was not as cuddly. I was to wait for the genetics team to call with an appointment, but to be honest, once I got home with her and life went on, I forgot all about them. I did listen to the doctors and all that they had to share with me about my daughter; maybe keeping her alive for the first six months of her life gave me strength, I don't know. What I did know is that we loved her; she needed us to be there and to be strong. I never treated her different from the way I treated my other children. She grew and learned as much and as fast as she could and, as long as she was happy, that was good enough for me.

Life changed a lot over the next year. Trina had started kindergarten and there were definitely ups and downs. She had a wonderful teacher's aide; her aide helped her follow through with school activities. Even though we had all met as a team with her new school principal and teachers, there were some misunderstandings. Trina's first teacher's aide was deaf. I don't know how it happened but I guess because she had had tubes put in her ears they assumed that Trina could not hear. She was wonderful with Trina; it was kind of funny in a ridiculous way. Here's a little girl who cannot speak much, but can hear, with a teacher who cannot hear and did not speak clearly. It did not take long for everyone to realize

Denise F. Loewen

this was not a good fit. Trina had a different aide the next week.

Things went well; she loved school, but I noticed changes happening that I could not explain. Her aggressive behavior started to show a little more, sometimes she would yell for no reason, and her seizures continued. In fact, they seemed to be getting worse. By this I mean they were longer and stronger and it was harder for me to get her back. After she would have a seizure she would be very tired and need to sleep.

The other huge changes were we became foster parents and we had a house fire. The damages were enormous; we lost everything and, of course had to find a new place. We couldn't find a house that was big enough for our family now that we had more children than just our own.

So, we moved to another town about an hour from the city we were living in. It was beautiful, and we found a house that was big enough for all of us. We were starting over again: new school, new doctors, and I didn't know anyone there. In the city I at least had my brother to help with Trina or my other children when I had to go to the hospital with her. When I think back now, it amazes me how the universe works. Little did I know at the time that I would end up meeting the doctor who would stick by us and save her life more than once. Miracles happen every day but, we are often too busy to take notice.

But living in a new town was not as hard as I thought it was going to be. All the kids loved it—the lake, the trails, even the bears that would come onto our deck and look into the bathroom window. Oh my God, what a different life. We didn't have a lot of furniture because of the house fire. People were so good to us, they donated clothes, beds, toys...it was all good. A new beginning.

It was the beginning of summer holidays; the kids were excited and met new friends. Trina loved to swim and there was a shallow indoor pool just down the street from us. Trina wanted to go there every day. We went for lots of walks on the trails by the lake. It was like a dream town.

The Tegretol Trina had been put on didn't seem to make any difference with her seizures. She still had them and they seemed to be getting stronger and longer. I was starting to realize that what the doctors had said about her outgrowing her seizures was not going to happen.

The summer was going well considering all her toys that she loved so much were all gone. She was such a trooper. It didn't matter what happened in life, she was always smiling and loving. But it was hard to figure out what was going on with her little body. There were so many changes for her. I had learned that stress could bring on seizures; lord knows there was enough of that—not just for her but for the whole family. The house we moved into was beautiful—the kids all had their own rooms, but something was not right for Trina. She did not like her bedroom and she wouldn't sleep in her bed anymore. She used to love sitting on her bed, doing puzzles and listening to her music. She was so good at puzzles it was amazing. The only way she would sleep in her bed was if I would lay with her. I'd have to wait for her to go to sleep, and even with doing that I would find her sleeping in front of the TV in the living room on the floor. The daytime hours were fine, she didn't seem to be afraid of the downstairs or being in the house. She just would not sleep in her bed. We did a lot of fun stuff. Trina loved physical activities—going to the parks, playing ball, and her favorite was being on the swing. This seemed to soothe her.

We met the new doctors in our town and they were both very nice. Other than her seizures Trina was a very healthy little girl. The doctors were very honest about not really having dealt with epilepsy before. Sometimes that's not a bad thing. These doctors seemed to listen to me more than the others that we had dealt with over the years. It was nice to be treated with respect; I missed that from our family doctor in Saskatchewan.

We finally received the call for us to take Trina to see the genetics team. We would be at the hospital for a few days. During this appointment they would do a head to toe assessment on her. It was very intense. We went through every day of her life and my pregnancy. They wanted to know everything about her. This took a few hours; there was a lot of information to share with them. First they did hours of verbal, physical, and occupational assessments.

Trina did well for the most part. I explained that I was seeing a bit of aggressive behaviour from her and this was not normal for her at all. Since Trina had been diagnosed with two syndromes, Noonan and Pierre Robin, the doctors also took pictures of her body and measured every inch of her. She was small for her age, but that was not unusual since she was so sick as an infant. They took x-rays of her bones and found that the Dilantin seizure medication she had been on had already started to change the bone structure in her face. This is something I was not told could happen. This made me very aware that I always needed to ask a lot more questions when she was put on any medication.

The fact that she was still having seizures was a concern to the doctors. While we were there they asked if they could bring in the neurologist to help them figure out what they could do about her seizures. Trina had another EEG and again they did not find any seizure activity. They took her blood to take levels of the Tegretol in her system. What they decided to do was to increase the Tegretol medication and add another medication. (I have tried to remember the name of it but, for the life of me, it is gone from my brain.) They felt this should help stop them for her.

At the end of the day, what we learned was that the doctors didn't really know any more than I did at that time. It would take some time for the results from her blood work to come back. They told us they didn't think she had Noonan syndrome, but the blood tests would tell them more. They said that she was developmentally delayed but felt that in time she could catch up. We did learn a few things but there weren't a lot of answers for anything. When I left there I felt that they had done all they could—they had seemed to be very thorough. They gave us numbers to call them if there were any more questions. All I wanted was for her seizures to stop and not get worse. I loved her so much, and we already had so many frightening times in her short life.

Again we went home with high hopes that Trina was getting the right treatment. It was always so wonderful to get home and be with all my kids. They were so strong and helpful with their little sister. The only thing I ever wanted was to be a good mom...no, I take that back, a great mom.

Once we got home and started her on this new medication, things went bad right away. In the morning I gave her the first dose and a few hours later she was yelling; it was a long day of her being agitated. She did not sleep that night and had more seizures than she had ever had. I didn't know what to do. Her seizures got so bad that I had to take her to the hospital. At the hospital they gave her some Valium. This calmed her down and she stopped seizing. I explained

Denise F. Loewen

that we had just been to her specialists and they had added a new medication. The doctors at the hospital called them to let them know what was happening with her. They said to take her off the new medication; they couldn't explain why she was having such a reaction, but it was best to stop it. Her seizures then stopped and I could take her home. I was glad they took her off the new medication. Trina's body reacting that way was very hard on her.

The summer was long. The kids missed all their friends they had in the city. It was amazing how many wonderful people we had met through school and daycare. The kids made friends quickly, and I was glad for that. I was so busy with the changes I was seeing in Trina. She had gone through a growth spurt during the summer. This was a positive thing. I was a little worried about her going to a new school. It was a lot of work to get everything organized. It wasn't like enrolling a regular child. I had to meet with the principal and teachers and explain Trina to them, trying to be positive about the things she was capable of and also talking about all the things she could not do. It's hard to talk about the negative things about your child. I was always a strong believer in concentrating on the good things in life and all the positive things that she had accomplished. It all went well. The staff at the school got to meet her before school started. I felt good about it and was not too worried.

I kept in contact with her neurologist; her seizures were getting noticeably worse and the aggressive behavior she had started showing was also increasing. A couple of weeks after the doctors had increased her Tegretol they increased it again. This did not sit well with me. The medication didn't stop her from seizing and it almost seemed like she was getting worse. Trina was tired from all the seizures she was having and was falling asleep during the day; this was not normal for her. When she slept is when she had the most seizures.

After the second increase Trina started to make clearing sounds in her throat. Every day it got worse; it was so bad that she couldn't talk without clearing her throat after each word. This was so frustrating for her—she would repeat words over and over again. Her sentences were two to three words long, but she couldn't even get these out. I called her neurologist and tried to explain what was going on. It was odd to me that they began to say that she could have a type of syndrome that causes kids to clear their throats. While I was on the phone Trina was trying to talk to me and couldn't get her words out. Instead of trying to explain what was happening I put the phone to her and got her doctor to listen to how she was sounding. I felt that because I didn't agree that she had another syndrome they just said they didn't really know what was happening and to just keep an eye on it. I also tried to tell them her seizures had gotten worse since her last increase in the Tegretol. They didn't feel that it was caused by the increase, but rather, that her body hadn't adjusted to it yet. I just didn't have a good feeling about it at all.

When your gut says there is something wrong, it's very important to listen to it. Wow, was my gut ever right.

A few days later I was living a real nightmare. I woke up in the morning; Trina had had a few seizures through the night. It was odd for her not to wake up with me, but considering she had had a rough night I didn't think too much about it. I gave the kids breakfast and kept checking on her. She was sleeping very soundly. It was almost noon so I decided to wake her up so she would eat something, I didn't like her going too long without fluids. When I tried to wake her up she didn't respond. I washed her face with a cloth and talked to her. I have to say that my stomach felt sick just remembering this to write it down. It felt like it was happening all over. She did not look like she was seizing by looking at her body, but when I pulled open her eyelids to try and get her to respond that's when I noticed her eyes were seizing. They were moving back and forth. It's something I had remembered when I was learning about different signs of epilepsy. I called her neurologist again and told them what was happening. They suggested that I get her to the hospital as soon as I could.

It was three-and-a-half-hour drive to the hospital and I couldn't take her myself. I managed to find a sitter for my other children and arranged a ride. I got there with her and sat in the emergency room waiting for a doctor to see her. By this time she had started to come around a little bit. When the doctor finally saw us, he took some blood work and told me to take her home. He said someone would call me at home and let me know what the blood work showed. I didn't even ask any questions—I was kind of stunned, I guess. I didn't think we would just be sent home. Even now it seems like it is impossible for it to have gone that way, but it did. I was so scared, leaving the hospital with her like that. On the way home she yelled most of the way. I felt bad for my friends who had driven us, but there was nothing I could do. It seemed like she had a headache, and was in pain. Usually if I sang to her it would calm her down, but nothing worked that day. It was a long drive home.

People, all people—family, friends, and even strangers—would want to help us when they saw Trina upset or having a seizure. They wanted to help, but never really knew how. I was always so grateful for the offers, but didn't even know how to let them help. For the most part we were just a regular family that had beautiful children with amazing souls.

Once we were home again, nothing really changed. Trina still had the throat clearing issue. She seemed to be okay from the seizure she had experienced. She was tired and agitated for most of the day and did not sleep well that night. She had more seizures through the night, but "normal" ones. Weird saying normal about a seizure, but they seemed to be part of her life now. It seemed like there were not many days that she did not have at least one. I just wanted them to find a medication that would stop them.

I was slowly getting to know our new doctors, but there was not a lot they could do for her. She didn't get sick very often, not the kind of sick that most kids get, like colds or flues. Within 48 hours of being home, the hospital called to say that they were very concerned about the results of the blood tests. They showed that her level of Tegretol was at an overdose level and that I needed to stop giving it to her immediately. This was the cause for her clearing her throat all the time. It was also the reason why she had gone into a coma state seizure. They assured me that because the clearing of her throat had not been going on for too long it should go away once the medication was out of her system. Once again the medication that was supposed to help her had made her sick. She could not be put on Tegretol ever again. If she was the doctor told me the clearing of her throat would come back. If this were to happen it may be with her forever. I thanked the doctor—yes I really did—once again I was just happy to have an answer to a problem that had nothing to do with her body but was caused by a medication. That might seem strange but all I could think was that knowledge as to the "why" was what was important. All I remember after that was holding her and telling her, "sorry," over and over.

Denise F. Loewen

It took about a week for the throat issue to go away, and her seizure frequency lessened. Trina seemed to do better when she was not on any seizure medication. Even though she still had seizures, they were less often and less severe. I'm so glad that I had the guts to disagree with the doctor on the phone when she said it was another syndrome that was causing her to clear her throat all the time. It was at this time that I started to question the medications. So far, every medication the doctors had given her made her sicker and had horrible side effects. I kept thinking about the EEG she'd had that didn't show seizure activity, but when they didn't find brain damage they came back to the epilepsy diagnosis. I didn't know what to think. I just didn't understand why the most popular medications for epilepsy made her sicker and didn't stop her seizures.

Next, Trina's eating became strange. She wouldn't eat anything with any flavor. She craved milk; she would prefer to drink milk than eat food. She would eat foods with very little taste, such as potatoes, cornflakes, plain chips, very bland vegetables, and fruits. When there is a drastic change in appetite in your child you definitely take notice. Trina was growing and this was great. In almost every aspect of her she was healthy. She very seldom got sick and she had beautiful skin, hair, and nails. She loved to play and for the most part was very happy and enjoyed playing and hanging out with her sisters and brother. The summer went on; Trina would soon be six years old. The funniest thing happened—Trina got hooked on super Mario. She didn't want to play but wanted the other kids to play and so she could watch. With five kids in the household, she could usually talk someone into playing for her. She loved her music and took a liking to decks of cards. She would sort them, sometimes by, numbers, sometimes by the colors. She would organize them in an order that only she understood. If anyone fooled around with her cards she knew and would sit down and organize them all again; she also knew if a card was missing. Even if she had more than one deck she still knew. It always amazed us. She also knew if a piece to her puzzle was missing before she would put it together. If one was misplaced she would search until she found it. Or she would have all of us looking for her. She was a lot happier and not so frustrated with her speech. I was so glad when the clearing of her throat had completely stopped. We were a happy family and she brought us closer together, that's for sure.

Denise F. Loewen

Learning to Question

It was time to get prepared for school. We had a meeting with the school to go over Trina's needs and to meet her new TA. I had asked for them to meet before school started—this would make it easier for both Trina and the TA. We had also agreed that a second year in kindergarten would be beneficial. That way she could be at school for a full school day. She was delayed and still very small for her age, so she would fit in with the younger kids much better.

But the changes that I was starting to see in her were showing up to a much larger degree. She would start screaming in class and would throw books around. The teachers didn't know how to deal with it so they would call me and I would pick her up. Sometimes I could just go to the school and spend some time with her and calm her down. I had no explanation for this change.

When she would have a seizure at school I would also have to pick her up. Sometimes things would be great for weeks at a time and then out of the blue she would have seizures and or be angry and yell. It wasn't anything people were doing; she could be sitting doing her puzzles by herself and just start yelling. Like I said before, Trina loved school. She would get up and get ready; put on her little backpack and off we would go. If I kept her home she would still want to wear her bag. She really loved her TA; she would say her name every day and talk about her on the way to school. Her classroom teacher was also awesome.

It was definitely a good place to live. I kept to myself for the most part of my days. Trina kept me busy and I was continually trying to figure out why she was changing so much. I kept telling her doctors, "This is not her." I know they didn't know what to think of me at first, but I didn't have time to worry about that. I think now that what probably helped me find answers for Trina is that I never worried about what people said or what they thought of me as a person after I left the room. When you have a child who relies on you every waking minute of every day, silly things don't come into play. I was getting to know the doctors in our new town better—I liked them and they listened to me. Even if they thought I was a little overwhelming, they did not treat me like I didn't know anything. I was already tired of getting the feeling from a lot of professionals that I was just her mom. I really came to rely on the doctors who listened and tried to help me find solutions to the changes that were happening to her.

Time passed, we tried to make every day as positive as possible. I knew things were getting harder at school. Trina would have fits of anger for no apparent reason. I didn't know what to think—she was getting worse and I couldn't figure it out. All I could do for the school was to be available to pick Trina up when it was too much for them. I totally understood. I also didn't want her at school if she was having a bad day.

Months went by, and then we received a call from the genetics team. They wanted to see us to talk about Trina's blood tests. I wanted to know over the phone but they insisted that they talk to us in person about the results. We would go to the big city once again to meet with them. I don't remember thinking anything about it. I was so focused on helping her in the now that tomorrow wasn't even on my mind. I had been to these meetings before; I was hoping they could help me figure out why she seemed to be changing so much. Little did I know that what they were going to share with us was going to affect how she was treated by the medical system for the rest of her life.

THINGS ARE NOT ALWAYS WHAT THEY LOOK LIKE FROM THE OUTSIDE

Off we went again to the big city for some more life-changing news. We decided to make it a family vacation. We would go to the appointment and then go visit friends and go camping. This was very exciting for the kids. We didn't get to go a lot of places; between work and Trina not being well we stayed pretty close to home. We did go camping and on day trips and she loved to be in the car. She was such a good traveler. We just had to make sure we were close enough to home and to hospitals and doctors. It was just our way of life—we all knew it and it wasn't a big deal. All the kids were so understanding when it came to their sister; they never complained when a trip had to be cut short or if we had to change our plans for Trina. This is what I call unconditional love—I don't like to brag, but that's one of the first things Trina taught us. She loved us no matter what we were going through.

This trip was scheduled for us and we just decided to take advantage of this appointment. First things first—we would get the appointment over with and then enjoy our vacation.

Not knowing what to expect when we got there, we went to the front desk to let them know we were there. Everyone was very nice to us; the receptionist took us to a large room. We were to wait there, she told us, and the doctors would be with us shortly. We had left her sister and brother with friends of ours, so we just had Trina with us. Thinking back, I remember always being so proud of my kids. Trina was so beautiful, she had a smile that would melt your heart and the most gorgeous long blonde hair—this was her trademark anyone who ever met her you would remember the little girl with the beautiful long blonde hair. It certainly makes me smile when I think about it. Anyway, we waited and soon doctors started coming in and introducing themselves. There were six, maybe eight, doctors. As they came in and the chairs began to fill up, I was getting a little nervous. I had no idea that there would be so many doctors. We had brought books and crayons for Trina so she was busy doing her own thing, sitting on the floor. She was very content and could keep herself busy. She did not understand that we were there for her. She never asked why, when, or what we were doing as long as she had her favorite things.

The meeting began and one of the doctors started to talk and to say he was sorry for the information they had to share with us about our daughter. I think at that moment I stopped breathing. I don't remember saying anything. I just nodded and listened. One at a time they talked about blood work and her genes and tried to explain that the syndrome that Trina was originally diagnosed with was wrong, she did not have Noonan syndrome but in fact had a syndrome called 3p minus. This was an extremely rare chromosome disorder and Trina was only the 11th child who had been diagnosed with it. This syndrome affected her third chromosome—the tip of this chromosome was missing. They did not know a lot about the genes that were in that missing piece, but it was going to make a dramatic impact on her development.

Denise F. Loewen

The easiest way for me to explain how my brain was working during all of this was that it was like in the movies when someone is getting extremely bad news and they are looking at the doctor but things aren't registering—you can see their lips moving but you're not even there anymore. They must have noticed the blank look on my face and it occurred to them that we should be asking questions. We took a break. Trina asked to go pee. I took her when we came back in the room they were all there waiting for us. Once again they start talking. One of the doctors was very apologetic and went on to tell me that my daughter would never talk, walk, or feed herself. She would never be potty trained or develop past infant stage. She would be extremely mentally handicapped and most likely be severely autistic. All the other children had heart and lung problems and did not grow physically. They also said all the other children had crippling scoliosis and that the other children never reached adulthood. They all passed away from kidney failure.

The only thing Trina had in common with the other children was they all also had seizures. They had the information on the other 10 children and said that we could have this information to take home. I was speechless listening to them and all the bizarre things they were telling me. Finally I found my tongue; I had to interrupt them before they went on any further. I looked around at these doctors who were specialists in their field. My exact words that came out of my mouth were: "I'm sorry, but I think you have the wrong family." I looked over at Trina coloring in her book and said, "That's Trina. She already does all the things that you said she would never do." I was stunned and shocked. I wish I had a stronger word but I don't think one exists. They looked over at Trina; she had asked to go pee; she was potty trained and had been since she was two. She walked, talked, fed herself and had been in school since she was three years old.

Now it was their turn to be speechless! They did not know that the little girl with us was Trina. They had thought she was one of our other children. They watched her play for a while and one of the doctors looked at us and said, "Well I guess there is nothing else we can share with you; she shouldn't be able to do any of the things." They also assured us that Trina did have the syndrome and they apologized for not knowing more about her.

How the conversation turned was incredible. Now they were asking me for information about Trina. I really didn't know what to tell them except we never treated her any differently than we did our other children. The proud mother came out of me fully. Trina was an amazing little girl and it showed more and more every day. After hearing what they had to say, I knew it more than ever. It took a little longer for her to catch on but once she learned something she had it. They asked if they could watch her closely and if we could keep them updated on her progress. We had no problem with that. I did talk to them about the changes I had started to notice. They didn't have any answers for me at that time, but said they would set up an appointment to do a complete assessment on her. By doing this they could help to make sure she received extensive therapies, such as speech, physio, and occupational. They explained that doing the assessment would help Trina receive these therapies in our area and school. This was exciting. We had been trying to get her therapy, but spots on waiting lists were all we got for her. When she did come up on the list it was for a very short time. There were so many kids waiting just like she was and it was hard to be angry about it.

Denise F. Loewen

ANGER FROM THE PAST HAS NO PLACE
WITH LOVE IN THE FUTURE

Once again we went home. We had made the best of our vacation. The kids had a wonderful time and we saw so many great things. We didn't dwell on what the doctors had shared with us about Trina. I do remember laughing a little, so many doctors in her short life and no one seemed to really know any more than I did. This gave me strength from within that is hard to explain in words. I guess "power" is the best word I can use.

I didn't realize it at the time, but as the years went by I got stronger and stronger. First, I had gained knowledge by reading and talking with other people. Second, I listened to doctors taking what fit for my daughter and putting the rest aside. I learned quickly that a university degree on a wall didn't always mean they knew more than I did about my daughter. Don't get me wrong, they definitely had more knowledge of the medical field and had access to much more information than I did, but I knew my daughter. Mother's intuition, a mother's bond, or a spiritual connection—you can call it whatever you want, I just knew I had it.

We waited again for the next appointment. Life went on as usual, at least as usual as things could be for our family. Trina loved school and loved to play; her new sport was basketball. She didn't understand the rules of the game but could get a basket almost every time. She had another growing spurt, which was great. She was finally starting to catch up to other kids her age. We moved to a different house (remember Trina did not like the house we were living in). We learned to pay attention to her feelings and when we went to look for another place to live we took her to the house first. She seemed to have a sixth sense about the energy around her. She loved the next house; she once again slept in her bed and loved to play in her room. It was so nice to see her listen to her music and spend calm time in her own space. It was nothing I did, it was just her feeling safe.

Even though Trina was growing and developing, something was still off. She would get angry and her eating was again changing. She was still having seizures, but they were not as bad as they had been when she was on medication—but they were still there. We went for a lot of walks, or I guess you could call them hikes. Living in the mountains you were always going either up or down. It was the perfect place to raise young children. In the winter there was tobogganing and skating on the lake, in the summer biking and walking. For the most of Trina's days she was happy and healthy. She learned how to ride a bike—her favorite was her Big Wheels.

Months went by and school started again. We'd had a great summer. Trina missed school and was so happy to go back. She loved her TA and had asked for her throughout the summer. Trina was in grade one that year and it would be her second year at this school, so the stress of being new was not an issue. Everyone knew her and loved her. We also had gotten to know the doctors in town a little better. Trina was not a sick child, so other than her seizures we really didn't see the doctors much.

Trina's seizures still scared me every time; my heart would miss a beat when I would hear the sounds she made that signaled she was starting to seizure. I didn't panic so much anymore and I felt comfortable that I was handling them the best that I could for her safety. Her TA was also more comfortable with her. There were signs to watch for, now that Trina was getting older it seemed like she could give us warning

Denise F. Loewen

before she would have a seizure. The two main signs were being agitated and repeating "Mom" over and over again. By then the school didn't call me every time she had a seizure. I still received a call if the seizure went on too long and then they would usually take her across the street to her doctor; I would meet them there. There really was nothing anyone could do but hold her and make sure she was safe and getting oxygen.

I started to recognize that Trina would seizure most when she was in pain. This could be a headache or stomachache. I could tell when she had a headache because her eyes would get glassy and her forehead would swell. She also started to have issues with her tummy. She seemed to be constipated more often. When she would have these pains her seizures would be worse, so bad that sometimes we would have to take her to the city hospital. This is where her pediatrician and neurologist came into our lives. They would be called when she went to hospital. It seemed the older she got the worse things became. There were more EEGs done and some seizure activity was found in the bottom part of her brain. This part of the brain controlled her vision and speech. This would explain why she was having difficulty speaking. She still only had three to four word sentences. There didn't seem to be any problems with her vision. Since she no longer took the Dilantin seizure medication she no longer needed glasses. I really wasn't listened to when I would try and explain that she had a headache or sometimes she hadn't gone to the bathroom for a few days. They did not seem to feel this would cause her to seizure. And this is where the 3p minus syndrome diagnosis begins to play a huge roll in her life.

The next few years went by with a lot of hospital stays and more doctors. There seemed to be no explanation for the huge changes in behavior and increase in seizures. I really hate to use the word behavior and my daughter in the same sentence. I always felt there was more going on with her than I could get her doctors to believe. Even though Trina was happy most of the time and played like every other kid there was a look in her eyes that told me there was more. Sometimes she would grab me and hang on so tight, and then something would switch and she would push me away. She had a need in her that only I could fill. Some days she would repeat, "Mom, Mom, Mom," over and over.

Her new pediatrician was very open about telling me she was spoiled and I needed to discipline her more. At first I didn't really say much, I would listen, be angry inside when we left his office and continue to search for what was really wrong with my daughter.

We had another appointment with the genetics team. They did another complete assessment on her. This covered every detail about her body and mind. Trina did not co-operate all the time when we were there. They measured her body and worked with her brain to see where she was developmentally. This was a very trying assessment. We were there with her for four days. She was getting very frustrated by the end of it all. Everyone was very nice to us when we were there, but it was also frustrating for me because I couldn't get any answers for my questions. I had given them all the information about her from the time I was pregnant. I wanted them to know that the frustrated little girl they were seeing was not who she was. I knew she didn't need to be disciplined, she was sick. I couldn't explain it and I certainly couldn't prove it. I just knew in my heart and my gut something else was wrong. I can feel the same feelings now. Writing this and sharing this with you I have a scream in my head that hurts. When you

Denise F. Loewen

need someone, anyone, to listen to you and they brush you off like you have no idea what you're talking about, it is the most helpless feeling in the world.

I would like to say now, if you're reading my daughter's story, there is a reason that this information came to you. If you are going through some of the same things that you have read about us, I want you to stop take a deep breath and don't give up. I'm not saying that the professionals that are in your life are wrong with the medical information they are contributing to your loved one's life, just make sure there is nothing left that needs to be considered. Remember when Trina was three months old I had asked if she could have an illness called pyloric stenosis and the doctor at the time wouldn't even consider it because she was not a boy. It turned out that was what was wrong, and a surgery fixed that problem for her. She could have developed much more quickly if she'd had it at three months old and not six months. I had the same gut feeling now seven years later. I may have gone on with life and I know that I was extremely grateful that she was alive and well. That doesn't mean that I forgot that I was right all along. I needed to stay strong for myself and for my daughter.

The questions that I had, I felt, should have had answers. Trina would get a swollen forehead when she had a headache. She was getting more headaches as she got older and the swelling seemed to not go away. When you touched her forehead it felt soft and like there was fluid under her skin. On her neck right under the base of her skull there was also the same puffy feeling. They did not have an explanation for this. The changes in her eating were also of concern to me. She started to have a gagging reflex with smells and tastes. Foods that she normally would eat were now making her gag so badly that I wouldn't even try to get her to eat them—these were foods with a strong taste or smell.

This is where it began. They didn't have any explanation for this because her syndrome was extremely rare and no one really knew much about it. The fact that Trina had progressed much further than any of the other 10 children, we were lucky that she had come so far. To tell you the truth, I really didn't put too much thought into the syndrome, 3p minus. She had already been diagnosed with Noonan syndrome and they were wrong about that. Her syndrome diagnosis was not an issue to me, her health was. From this assessment Trina's diagnosis would change from being delayed in development to being mentally retarded. I believe this was mostly to do with her frustrated outburst and the lack of inclination she had toward following orders.

At the end of the assessment was a meeting with the team that had seen her during this stay. There was not a lot of information—Trina was small for her age, she was delayed mentally, but physically she seemed to be fine. She didn't have any of the medical problems that the other children had; her heart, kidneys all her organs were very healthy. I knew that from when she had her surgery on her stomach and woke up before they were done stitching her up and the surgeon was very impressed with how strong her heart was. They also wanted to put her on a new seizure medication called clobazam. We were told it was a new medication with very few side effects. We agreed to this even though the last medications hadn't stopped her seizures—as Trina's health was our first priority, we were willing to try another one.

I took a deep breath and held her close. They would send all the information to her doctors in our hometown and to her pediatrician and neurologist so they would have as much information about Trina as possible and be better able to help.

When I received the letter from them weeks later, it read that Trina was a beautiful little six-year-old girl with a behavioral problem. My heart stopped. That's what they came up with. This letter was sent to all her doctors. I can't even remember what the rest of the letter said. And really, this one sentence was the only one that would affect Trina's life in any way. The rest of the information was irrelevant.

Things just kept getting harder and harder. Trina did fairly well on the new medication, but her seizures were never completely gone. What I felt (and still feel in my gut) is extremely hard to put into words but I'll try my best. We went on with our daily lives as best we could.

We moved once again to another house in the same little town. It was perfect—right across the street from the school, and there was park in our back yard. I couldn't have asked for more if I had ordered it myself. Trina went to school every day. She loved walking to school with the other kids. We were working on teaching her safety, as she had no fear of anything. She did not understand the dangers of life such as cars or the lake. Trina had to have supervision 24/7. I never really thought this as an issue. I worked at home and we took her wherever we went. We also had her sisters and brother to help keep an eye on her. They loved her so much and never turned her down if she wanted to go to the park or over to the school to play. Trina made our family very close; my kids were not selfish children and always stuck up for their little sister.

Trina's—I'm not sure what to call it—aggressive behavior was continuously getting worse. She wanted to be close like she was used to, but when I hugged her she would push me away. Or she would pull me close, then get upset and push me away. It was like she didn't know how to handle whatever she was feeling. Trina didn't have a good vocabulary and really only spoke of the things in life that interested her. She couldn't tell you if she was in pain. We all had to learn to read her body gestures to know what we needed to do for her.

We had a family support worker come into our lives. She would take Trina on outings once a week and try to get a handle on her so-called behavior. She was there to help our family interact differently and improve our discipline of Trina. I was grateful for her help and input, but I just didn't agree that it was behavior. Trina really liked her and enjoyed their outings, but nothing we tried helped. This was hard for me. I kept saying something is wrong—she doesn't have a discipline problem. Over and over again I would tell all the professionals in her life that she was sick. More and more Trina was confused. Things that she normally liked to do and entertained her weren't working. She was still comforted by the motion of swinging. Her school actually put a swing in their classroom to help soothe her when she was upset. They tried so hard to help and she was still progressing. She was learning how to read and print. This is what made it so hard for me to think that her problem was discipline. She didn't get angry when she was told no, it was unexpected, during times when she was doing her favorite things.

Being on seizure medication was a tough call. It may have helped with some of her seizures by slowing down the brain activity, but it also slowed down her body functions. Her intestinal tract was being affected. She had an extremely hard time moving her bowels. When I would tell her pediatrician that she wasn't going everyday and it seemed to affect her mood, he didn't agree. The explanation that I got was that

Denise F. Loewen

it was normal for special needs children to only have a bowel movement a couple times a week. I don't know about you, but all the research I've done says it's not good for your body to have irregular bowels. I wanted to believe this, but something in my gut told me, "No way."

I once again had something new to learn about. I read about the intestinal tract and asked questions. When I would take her to our family doctor they were very honest about what they knew about her syndrome and how it was affecting her. We spent a lot of time with her pediatrician—not that we would go to him, but when Trina ended up in the hospital for seizures he would be called. It was during this time that I started to notice her seizures were worse when she seemed to be in pain. When I would mention her tummy, the doctors would order x-rays. These always showed that she had lots of gas in her intestines, and, at times, a lot of stool.

I didn't know what to do for her; she was not just agitated but actually screaming and she would hit and throw things. The pediatrician decided that she needed to be on medication for her behavior. When your child is screaming, can't sit still and is hitting you, it is hard to say no. I also wanted to do everything I could to help her. I didn't know, so I was willing to try almost anything. So new medications were added. Reperidone and valproic acid were what he felt she needed to calm her down. I'm ashamed to admit this but I tried it for a few weeks. Now you need to know that Trina was very active, she had been potty trained by the age of two and half and she had started to wet her pants and she would pee the bed. Finally I couldn't stand it anymore.

With this medication the hardest thing to see was that she would just sit and drool. Yes, she was calm, but there was no life in her. I took her to see her pediatrician to show him how bad it was. We were sitting in the room waiting for him and she was sitting beside me like a zombie. She wasn't talking anymore and was not interested in the things she used to enjoy. He walked in, looked at her drooling and said, "I see she's doing much better." I almost threw up. I couldn't believe that this was "better." I told him I wanted her off the new medication he had put her on. I wanted him to understand I'd rather her be screaming and hitting me than the way she was on the meds. At least she was telling me that something was wrong, and she needed me to help her. This did not fit for me at all. I guess he didn't agree because he thought she was just spoiled and not sick. He was not happy with me at all. It amazes me (now that I have more time to think about all of this) that he never touched her during our visits. I would talk, he would disagree, and that was the visit.

One day, after just getting home from a long drive, I pulled into the driveway and a car pulled up behind me. I didn't know who this was. Getting Trina out of the car was a challenge. She was not well, so I had taken her for a drive. The person who had come introduced herself and told me she was from mental health. She was asked to come and meet us to see if she could help with Trina. That was fine with me, at that moment my concern was getting her in the house as calmly as possible. She was still small for her age and at eight years old I could still carry her. We got in the house and I told the lady to make herself at home and that I would be right with her. I had Trina in the house and she was lying on the floor in the hallway. She was screaming and wanted to go back into the car. I lay down beside her and rubbed her back and that calmed her down for a while. She went to the couch and lay down. Now I was able to sit and talk with this lady who was there to help me. She had been referred by Trina's

Denise F. Loewen

pediatrician. The first thing she told me was that I should not give my daughter any attention when she is throwing a tantrum. I should be putting her in her room for some time out without using any words. Giving her positive attention is just encouraging her to behave the way she is. I looked at her and I couldn't breathe.

A thought came to me and I said it out loud, "You don't know anything about my daughter! How dare you come into my home and tell me not to give my sick daughter attention. She is not having a tantrum. She is sick."

I told her I was wasting her time and she was wasting mine, so would she please leave. I was shaking when she left; I was appalled that Trina's pediatrician would send someone to my home to tell me how to discipline my daughter. Whether I was right or wrong, that was no way to come into my home and talk about my daughter without even having a conversation with me or asking me some questions to get a better idea of what we were going through. That was that. I spent the rest of the day comforting my daughter the way she needed to be comforted.

Trina's screaming would sometimes go on for so long that driving in the car was the only way to calm her down. Once I started to do this for her the more she wanted to be in the car. I would drive and sing to her. I kept promising that I would make her better. I cried for her. Her behavior was getting so bizarre, and it scared me that I couldn't figure it out. The answer from the most knowledgeable person, her pediatrician, was to give her stool stimulants to compensate for the seizure medication slowing down her system. It did make sense to me at the time. Added to the stimulant was mineral oil. She was so sick; it was clearly not working. Back to the doctor. The answer was to increase the amount I was

giving her. I tried it for a few days but it produced screaming and more screaming. This was not a "behavior," it was a
scream of pain. The only thing that stopped the screaming
was the seizures.

Finally, when I knew she could not take this anymore, I
took her to one of our family doctors. I remember sitting in
his office with him explaining how much pain she is in; her
skin was starting to turn gray. I knew her body was being
poisoned. I was no doctor, but just looking at her I knew that
it was not good. She had stopped screaming and was sitting
in her chair rocking back and forth. Our doctor was honest
about not knowing what to do and he called a specialist and
explained what was.

The specialist said to stop giving her the stool stimulant
and the mineral oil; if she had a blockage this would not move
it. I'll never forget this as long as I live. We had a small diag-
nostic center in our little town; he told me to go there and he
would meet us. He was going to give her an enema to loosen
her stool. I had never experienced this before and really had
no idea what was going to happen. What I did know was that
my little girl was extremely sick and something needed to
be done now. He arrived as he said he would and gave her
an enema. At first nothing happened. A few minutes later
I took her to the bathroom and she started going. My poor
baby smelled like something had died in her, she pooped and
pooped; her poor doctor couldn't handle the smell and had to
leave the building. I'm not kidding—she cleared the building.
When she had finally stopped I took her home.

She slept for three days and the whole time her poor
little body drained stool. The toxins were coming out of her
pores. I was sick. As many times as we had taken her to the
hospital and she had x-rays, it didn't occur to anyone there

Denise F. Loewen

that this should have been done for her weeks ago. Once her body had gotten rid of the blockage I did everything I could to keep it from happening again. Once again, my reading and understanding how the body works was what prevented this from repeating this kind of thing. Because her intestines had been stretched from the blockage it was now going to be even harder to keep her bowels clean. I did learn that the bowels would heal themselves, but to do that you have to have clean bowels for them to heal. This was to prevent formation of a pocket that would collect stool that would normally pass.

What I learned from this was that I did know my daughter better than anyone else. I should have been more aggressive myself. I was her voice because she couldn't talk enough to tell them what was happening to her. When your child is non-verbal your voice and your knowledge is sometimes all they have. Again, we had gotten through a very rough time for her. I just wanted this to be the end of her pain. After this I let her pediatrician know that he would no longer be my daughter's doctor. A vet would have treated her with more respect. Once again I felt that a miracle had to happen for us.

Every Step Leads to Miracles

Many people in our lives had suggestions for me. I listened to every one of them. I took what I needed for her and put the rest somewhere locked in my brain. This didn't mean that I didn't appreciate all the advice, but it didn't all fit. Most people were very helpful. I got my strength from my dad. He was a wonderful man, raising five kids on his own. He had a lot of knowledge that he shared with us kids. When I felt like I couldn't do it, I would think of my Dad and how hard he had it back in the day when single dads were very few and far between. He taught me how to be a great parent. One of the quotes I remember him saying to me when I was a kid was, "You can't learn anything new with your lips flapping. You learn by listening." I don't think I understood the meaning of this until I became a mother and had to learn from and listen to so many people, people who I would not have been in my life if my daughter hadn't been sick. For that, Dad, I am forever grateful.

I feel that I made the right choices and picked the right things to apply to Trina's life. One of the best decisions I made was to listen to a person who advised me to see a naturopath. They tend to look at their patients as a whole and don't separate the mind, body, and soul. I found a naturopath who would change Trina's life. He had answers to some of the questions that the doctors couldn't answer for me. It was amazing experience for her. She would ask to go to see him. He relieved her headaches and he helped me get a handle on her bowels. The swelling on her forehead and behind her neck was from migraine headaches. He put her on herbal medication to help her liver function better and this helped her bowels work better. He helped her body as a whole and connected things that she was struggling with and didn't blame me for spoiling her and not teaching her with discipline. It's not that she didn't have rule—I expected the same from Trina as I did all my other children. He started by working on her skull to relieve her headaches. This really did work. Trina was getting to a point where she didn't like to be touched, but she loved to go to get her treatments from him.

There was much more I learned from Trina's naturopath that changed so many things for us. He taught me how to massage her head to relieve headaches between visits. He was very supportive with me as a parent; he kept my self-esteem up so I did not get down on myself. I could tell that her headaches were much less intense. Trina started to shove her pillow into her mouth when she seized. Her naturopath explained this was a way she had discovered on her own to help relieve the pain of her headaches. Putting pressure on the roof of your mouth does this.

Kids like Trina had a sixth sense about them—they naturally now how to do things without the input of others. Trina showed me this about herself many times throughout her life. Much of the time the things that took me forever to learn about her she was already doing herself. The first significant issue she had was the Pierre Robin syndrome she had been diagnosed with when she was only months old. This was a bone structure problem that affected her jawbone. It gave

Denise F. Loewen

her an overbite that made it hard for her to chew her food properly. As she grew the bone structure of her face did get worse. Her naturopath had a totally different explanation for Trina's bone structure. I was in labour with her for three days before they finally did a C-section. Having contractions for this amount of time was hard on her. Because she started to come down the birth canal, it squashed her head. This changed the bone structure of her head. Normally, this would have been looked at when the child was born, but thinking about her birth now I suppose that her other issues took precedence, such as not being able to breathe on her own and not being able to contain her body heat. The differences that I noticed with Trina's facial features compared to my other two children when they were born was explained to me by her doctors then that it was because she was premature and most premature babies had a more swollen look to them. This would correct itself as she grew and gained weight. It never did. There were so many other things that I couldn't put together. I learned that all things about the body affect every part of the body. I needed to see every detail as a part of a whole, otherwise how could I expect her doctors to?

So he started to work on manipulating her facial bones with his hands. It was amazing to watch. Trina was so comfortable with him and she always looked and felt better when we left. For months Trina saw him, at first it was only once a week, then she started to ask to see him in-between visits, so I stared to take her twice a week. The difference in her appearance was unbelievable. Her jawbone was so different that her overbite was decreasing. She was able to chew much better and she did not breathe through her mouth. By lifting her cheekbones her appearance started to change; she began to look like she should have from birth. Her nasal cavities were opened up so she could breathe through her nose. This made a world of difference for her.

After about eight months of having these treatments done I had to take Trina for a dentist appointment. She'd had x-rays done on her face before and at that time I was told she would need surgery to correct the problem with her bite. When her dentist saw her after the treatments from the naturopath he couldn't believe this was the same kid. He compared her mouth to the x-rays they had done when she was younger. Not only did she not have to have surgery to correct her jawbone, but she would not even need braces.

This was the most amazing news for us, for her. A breakthrough! I would even call it a miracle. Never did I think that so much could be done for her with the touch of gentle hands. I learned as much as I could from him. He was willing to teach me anything I wanted to learn. Her naturopathic doctor was getting up in years—Trina was actually his last patient. He was retiring but continued to see her for as long as he could. I was eager to learn as much as I could so I could continue to help her myself.

Another issue that he found was her spine had a slit curve. This was a problem that all the other children with her syndrome had—crippling scoliosis. I was so worried about her and how not getting these treatments was going to affect her. She had improved so much and he had given us so much hope. I just prayed I had learned enough. After he had seen her for the last time, I did get names from him of other naturopaths; the problem was he was the only one that specialized in the skull. I had no idea how difficult it would be to find another naturopath who could do for her what he did. I thank him with all my heart for the time he spent with my Trina.

Denise F. Loewen

Always keep an open mind to all new paths in life—don't be afraid of the unknown

I was much more aware of how doctors, teachers, and just people in general, looked at Trina as a human being. I think for some doctors it's not about the person with a beautiful soul and a journey to travel in this life, but more often they see the illness or the challenge and not the person. When they have to deal with a special needs child with problems they cannot identify, they tend to forget they are beings with feelings and love to give to the world. I know some of them missed this completely. When I was so persistent with getting her healthy, they would tell me that she could not be fixed, that I needed to accept the fact that she was handicapped. It seemed no matter how I tried to explain how it really was, they did not get it.

I loved my children with all my heart. I loved each one of them for who they were and what good they brought to my life and the lives of everyone they met. Trina had a special bond with others. Her teachers had a different part to play in her life. They understood that I wanted Trina to enjoy life, learn, and be the best person she could be. We all worked together to help her accomplish these things and all I wanted them to do was to follow her lead. I will be forever grateful to the teachers who understood this and loved her for who she was. Teaching her through music was the best way for her to learn. She could sing complete songs, but could not speak a full sentence. I also learned to work with them as well. Each one of her teachers brought something different to her life. She loved them, and they felt that. Trina had as much to teach others as they had to teach her. The people who understood that grew with her. Some people looked at her in awe and others felt sorry for her. I never felt sorry that she was special needs, but embraced her for who she was. I just never understood why her doctors overlooked any possibility that she may be sick and not just look at her as being handicapped.

Photos

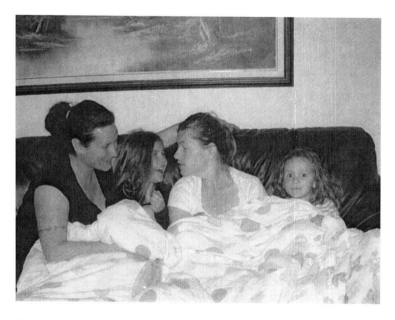

Trina with Jackie (sister), Annabella (niece), Pixie (niece). They love their auntie Trina so much. They would do puzzles and she made them laugh. This was after Trina's gallbladder surgery. So much of her life had been wasted being sick. She loved life and her family so much. She just LOVED.

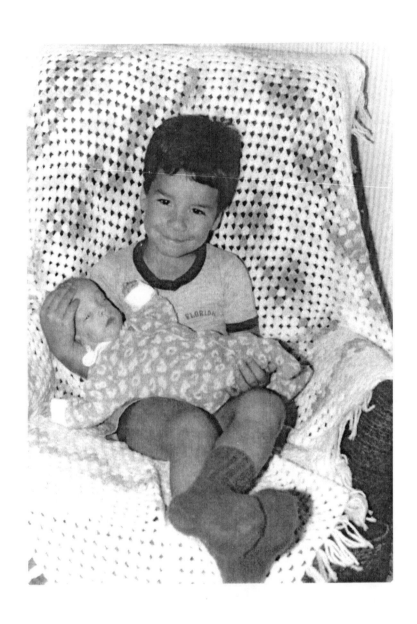

Denise F. Loewen

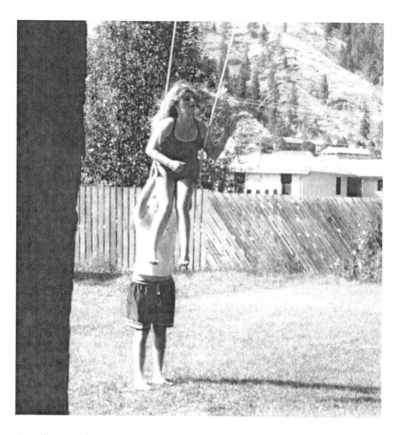

Jonathon pushing Trina on the swing. Trina would swing for hours. It would calm her down when she was stressed and in pain.

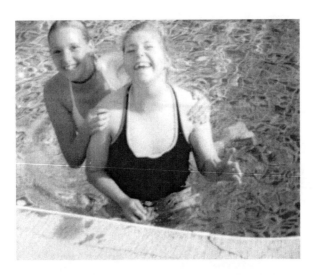

Trina and her cousin Megan. Trina loved to swim. It was the best therapy for her when she lost the use of her right side due to sizing.

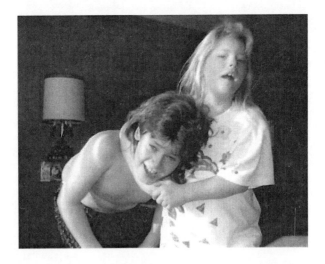

Trina and her brother Jonathon. Trina loved to play with her big brother. Jonathon spent a lot of time hanging out with Trina. She was always a big part of his circle of friends.

Denise F. Loewen

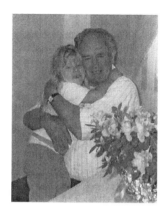

Trina at age 6 with her Grandpa. They were very close. Grandpa cried many tears when his little baby granddaughter would seizure. Trina's grandpa was one of very few people that were not afraid to help me with her when she was born. He was there for me in many ways, too many to count.

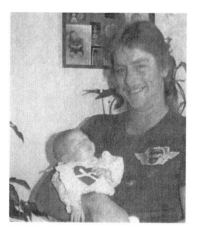

Trina's Uncle Dean. He was always so close to Trina. It was to Uncle's to spend over nights so Trina could have a break from home. She knew exactly were he lived.

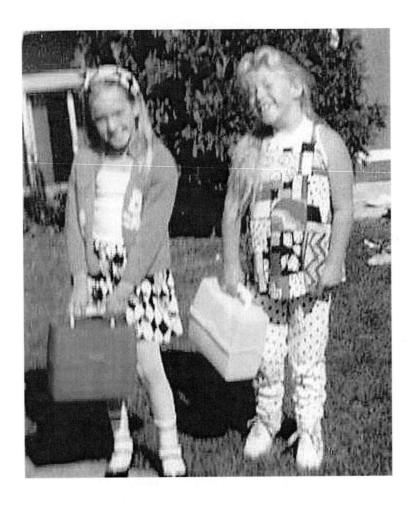

Trina with her cousin Megan. First day of school for both of them. They were so close. Trina had just started to show outbursts of frustration. Everyone has enough Vitamin B12 in their bodies from birth to keep them healthy for 5 years. Trina had just turned 6 years of age. Up until the age of 6, Trina had never shown aggressive behaviour. That was my argument with Doctors. She was not spoiled as they tried to tell me. She was always such a happy and calm child.

Denise F. Loewen

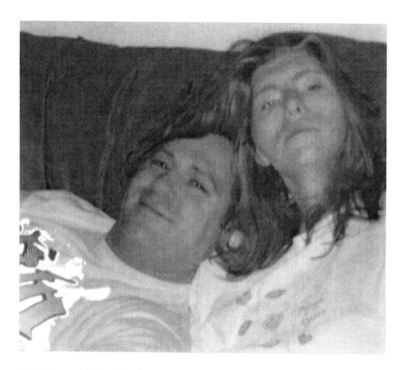

Relaxing with Tom (brother in law). He could always calm Trina.

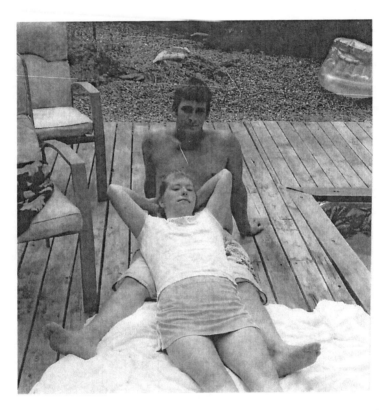

Trina and Jonathon (brother). Trina would sleep while Jonathon stood still. That's LOVE.

Denise F. Loewen

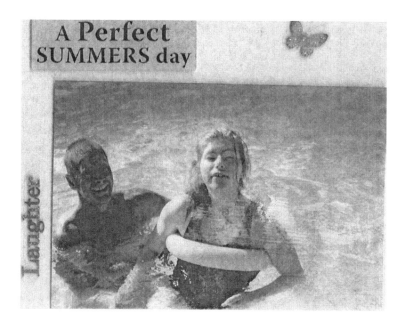

A Perfect SUMMERS day

Laughter

Trina and Uncle Dean. Trina loved to swim. Good therapy for her body and mind.

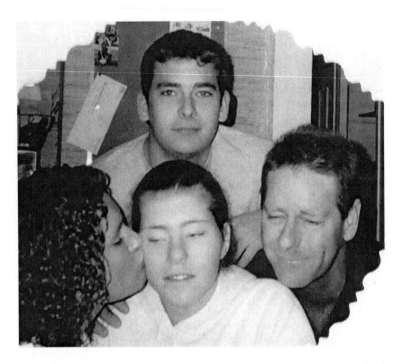

You can feel the love and see the relief in everyone's eyes. Trina had been given back to us. This is how she felt for exactly one year after her vitamin b12 shots. One year of pain free life. Seizure free for one year. Trina would ask to see her doctor for her shots. He got a big hug every time.

Denise F. Loewen

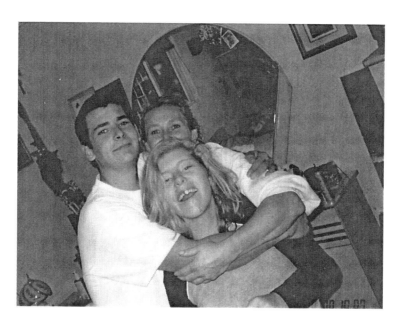

You can feel the love and see the relief in everyone's eyes. Trina had been given back to us. This is how she felt for exactly one year after her vitamin b12 shots. One year of pain free life. Seizure free for one year. Trina would ask to see her doctor for her shots. He got a big hug every time.

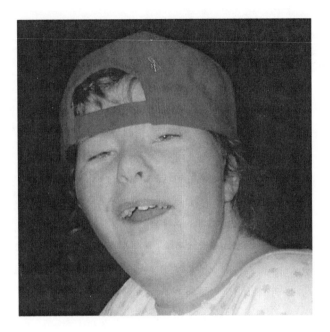

This picture was taken when Trina had just turned 17 years old. You can see how swollen her face and body are. It was shortly after this that her body shut down. Trina did not like to be touched.

Denise F. Loewen

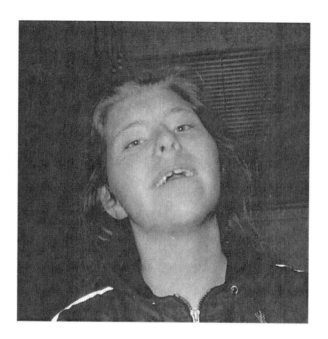

The gagging look on Trina's face was how she felt most of the time before the vitamin B12 shots started. Smells and tastes of foods made her feel like this. This went away after she received the shots.

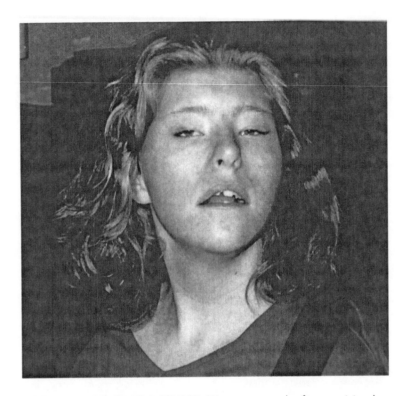

ONE OF MY FAVORITE PICTURES. Trina one month after receiving her vitamin B12 shots. Trina was back in school and had not had a seizure since she started getting the shots. She was so happy and never again showed any aggression.

Denise F. Loewen

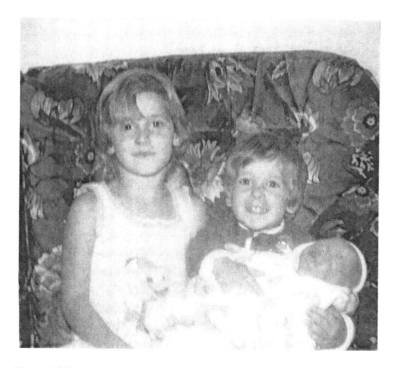

Trina with her sister, Jackie, and her brother, Jonathon age 2. Two very proud siblings. The three of them remained close to each other. Trina's protectors as she grew up.

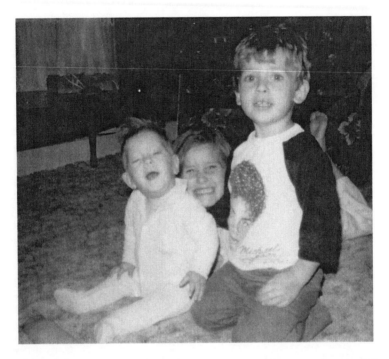

Trina almost 1 year old. Trina's eyes are not opening the way they should. She has started growing since her surgery at 6 months. So much hope. Trina is catching up with weight and physical abilities. Her sister and brother never lost their connection with Trina.

Denise F. Loewen

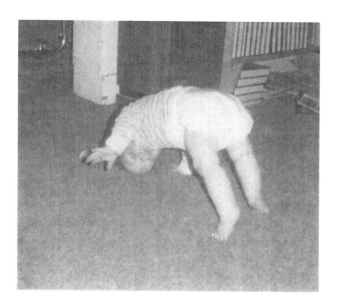

Trina started to look at the world upside down. She did this, I believe, because she could see clearer this way. After her eye surgery, she stopped doing this. She would laugh so hard when she was upside down; it would make her fall over.

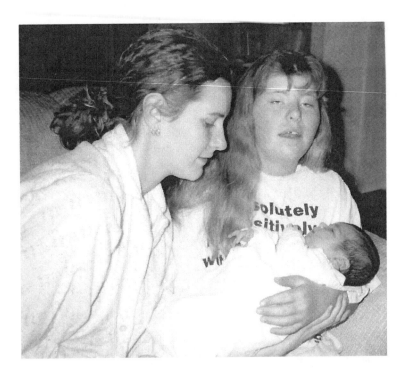

Trina with her sister, Jackie, and niece, Keira. You can see Jackie is having to hold Trina's arm for her. She has started to lose her body control at this age. Shortly after this, Trina seizured so often that she couldn't walk on her own and stopped talking. The only thing she continued to say was MOM MOM.

Denise F. Loewen

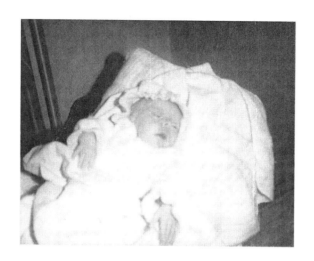

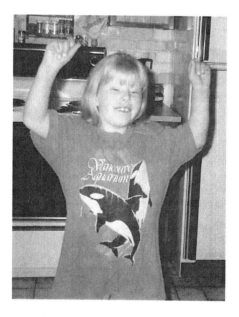

Trina, age 10. Trina's body is starting to swell. It was at this age until she was 17 years old that she had migraine headaches. She was always so strong and proud of herself. She brought so much joy to our family. Trina loved music and loved to dance.

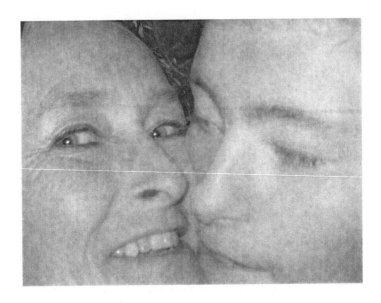

Trina and mom.

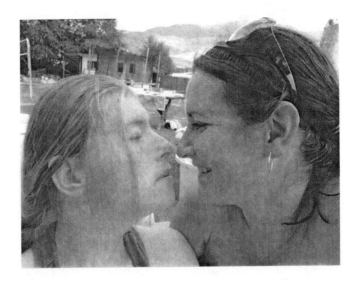

Trina and mom.

Denise F. Loewen

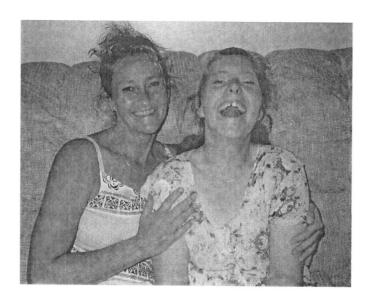

Trina and mom.

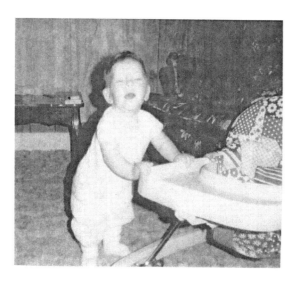

Trina at 1 year of age.

Mommy, Please Don't Listen To Them   107

Being Strong to be Heard

The huge spiritual awaking I am about to share is more about me than it is about Trina. If I close my eyes I can put myself right back there like it is just happening. When I am in survival mode and there seems to be no end to it, I will go and go like there is no stopping me. It's like the mom who lifts the car off her child. No one knows where that strength comes from; it's just love from a higher power that gives you the strength—divine power. That is what I believe to be true. I always knew it in my heart. What I'm going to share now some may call a dream, but to me it was a vision.

I'm in a room, there are four of us. We are playing cards, with friends. Everyone is talking to each other except me. I'm listening to the voices but it is like they are in a distance. The words fade out, and all I can hear are voices. I get up from the table we are sitting at. No one seems to notice that I have gotten up. I look at them as if they can't see me. I walk toward a door and it opens. I can still hear the others talking but can't make out what is being said. I'm through the door and it's dark, very dark, the voices stop; it's like they were never there. The darkness doesn't scare me. I'm just standing there looking toward a light in the distance. I know that I'm alone but it doesn't feel like it. I walk toward the light. I can hear humming. It's a beautiful sound. It makes me feel calm and relaxed. When I get to the light I feel like I have entered another space and time. I'm in a room; at first it's so bright I can't see anything, I can only hear the humming. A sense of peace washed over me like I have never felt before. My eyes adjust to the brightness of the room; across the room I see two images. They were not facing me, they were standing side by side. Both were wearing long white flowing gowns, to the floor. There was a glow of white energy all around them. One was tall with the strongest of energy, the other shorter. It was like looking through a thin fog. I couldn't tell you who they were and I don't even remembering wondering. I was just okay. I felt warm and welcome. I walk up behind them. The taller, I'll call her a lady, was the one humming, the smaller one was standing beside her. Neither one looked over at me as I approached them. I knew they knew I was there. I reach them and I'm now standing beside the smaller girl. I look over at them. It's Trina and an angel. I at once know that the angel is Trina's guardian angel. Without words, the spiritual connection is so strong I feel like I'm part of them. We are standing at a beautiful counter; her guardian angel is washing crystals and handing them to Trina. Trina is drying them with a soft cloth. She is so gentle and careful with these crystals. She's laying them on a white cloud that seems to be covering the counter. I felt so at peace, as if we were one. There were no words spoken—there was no need for human words. It felt like I was there for a million lifetimes. Trina looked over at me and smiled. I opened my eyes and I was back in the room with my friends, they were still talking and playing cards as if I never left. I looked back at the door, which had now closed and started crying. I wanted to go back. This is how my vision ends.

Denise F. Loewen

I lay in bed knowing that what I had experienced was Trina showing me that she was ok. Her guardian angel was always with her. I believe this with all my being that she was there for both of us. This vision will keep me on track with her. I never knew it was possible to feel more connected to her than I already was, but I did. To this day I can close my eyes and get right back there where I felt so safe and loved.

TO SEE AN ANGEL, YOU MUST SEE ANOTHER SOUL. TO FEEL AN ANGEL, YOU MUST TOUCH ANOTHER'S HEART. TO HEAR AN ANGEL, YOU MUST LISTEN TO BOTH.
—AUTHOR UNKNOWN

Strength, power, knowledge, guardian angels...if a family ever needed all of these it was our family. The next years would put us to the test. I became a single parent; this was the best for my children. It's hard to be in a relationship and not work as a team. I was terrified at the beginning, but soon realized I was fine. I always devoted my life to my kids, so that was not different. After the school year ended, I moved back to the city with my kids. We were happy, as happy as we could be. We all had our ups and downs, and sticking together was a huge part in our healing. After we moved I realized that one good parent was better than two bad parents. Of course there were highs and lows; there was anger from not under-standing why things go the way they do. I was so proud of my kids for sticking together and supporting each other. It was because of their love and compassion that I was able to care for Trina the way I did.

Living back in the city, it was all good. I found a house with a beautiful back yard, right down the street from the school.

The kids loved the yard. Trina spent a lot of time playing on the swing. Celebrating her ninth birthday, I couldn't believe how the time had gone by. I was still full of hope and faith that life would treat her well better. With my whole heart I always felt that when you do good things, good things would come back to you.

When we have lack of knowledge we sometimes complicate things unnecessarily and miss the simple answers. Trina's syndrome complicated the hell out of her life. The diagnosis complicated and confused the doctors who were suppose to help me keep her healthy. Fighting for her health against a diagnosis was one thing, but fighting professionals and a diagnosis for years just broke my heart and shattered my belief in a system that was supposed to be there to help and heal. I was definitely on survival mode; I didn't realize this during these next years of Trina's life, but you never do when you're in it.

New school, new life...so much to take care of and organize. The school was great; they were very open and responsive to Trina's needs. We were able to meet her new TA before she started school. We both really liked her. She was kind and gentle.

Most days I was thankful for all that I had, and other days I just wanted to scream at the universe for Trina's life being so hard. It just didn't make any sense to me. The doctors said she was perfectly healthy. They could never find anything wrong with her, but yet she was so sick. Since her naturopath had retired, I tried to do all the things he taught me. Things were getting worse for her. It seemed like every month her health got worse. Her seizures started to change—she didn't have seizures often when she was awake, but when she went to sleep they would come on strong. The seizures turned into

Denise F. Loewen

"grand mal" seizures. Trina still loved physical activities such as swimming, jumping on the trampoline, and playing ball. Her days were filled with school and playing at home. Even when I felt she should stay home she would get ready for school and put on her backpack wanting to go. It was only a block from the school, but sometimes we didn't make it that far. Things would change for her so quickly—one minute she would be laughing and singing and the next, screaming and as though she couldn't stop. That's when I would turn around and take her back home. The days went on like this all year. The doctors increased her seizure medication as she grew and her seizures became worse. She was still on the clobazam during this period of her life.

I had to stop writing for a few days. Writing Trina's life experiences have took me back to a place in her life that I had thought I had put behind me. I have always had the strength to forgive and move on. Being grateful for the times that I figured out what was making Trina sick was what kept me moving forward with our lives. I never dwelled on who was to blame or on the mistakes that were made that caused my daughter to suffer so unnecessarily. I made a few mistakes myself and wanted to be forgiven. I was able to do that. I now realize that I needed to go on being the parent that my children needed me to be.

Trina's difficulties continued around the clock: she was special needs with mental challenges, non-verbal, and very sick. It took all my strength to not only take care of her, but also be her speech therapist, occupational therapist, and her advocate with the school and health systems. She did get a few months of speech and occupational therapy before the age of seven. I knew she would not get the therapy that she needed so I took a speech therapy course myself to help her every day, not just once or twice a month. Because she was now in the school system she was put at the bottom of the list for all therapies. She also didn't qualify for services in the system because she was labeled mentally challenged and not physically challenged, therefore she was deemed unteachable. This was not the case and I knew it. Her TAs were very understanding as to how I felt. I can only hope that this has changed over the years. The older a child gets the further down the list they go as the younger children have top priority. I do understand why this is how it works, but doesn't make it fair. I learned everything I could from the people who worked in the system. They were all good people and it wasn't their fault that the system—well the system sucks. Yeah, that's definitely one of the choice words I can think of.

School was my relief. The days that she was at school were when I could take the time to learn and research as much as I could. I knew my daughter was sick and because she had been diagnosed with a syndrome that was so rare and no one knew anything about it, I was on my own. I had to convince doctors and teachers that I was not just an over-protective parent, that I really did know a few things about my daughter. I was always a very rational person; I had lived through many rough times myself as a kid and felt I was a survivor not a victim. I worked hard, loved my job, and was very grateful for who I had become.

Not only did I have to hold my head high and show the world that my daughter deserved every chance there was to provide her with a happy and healthy life, but keep my wits about me will doing so. There were many times when I would walk out of a doctor's office with Trina screaming and hitting and thanking them for their time, while what I was really feeling was that I wanted to scream with her and yell at

Denise F. Loewen

them for not listening to me. I would put her in the car and sit there sometimes not able to drive away. I would take deep breaths and calm her down as much as I could so I could drive safely. Telling her over and over again, "I'm so sorry Trina. I'll figure it out, I promise." I must have promised her a thousand times.

Trina started to swell—her body looked like if you poked her with a pin she would pop. Because of this drastic change in her appearance, it looked like she wasn't being fed properly. I was sent to nutritionist to teach me how to feed her better. I went, even though I knew I was feeding her healthy food. I did learn new things—even if it was only one thing that I had not learned on my own, it was worth it. Most doctors who had the privilege of working with her certainly did not agree that I knew what I was talking about. They said over and over there is nothing physically wrong with her. Drugs were their answer to almost everything. I disagreed. My reply was that she was sick. Our family doctor would listen to me; he would look for anything he could find. He even did tests over and over again thinking there was a mistake or that maybe something had changed with her. I will admit he didn't find anything that could give me an answer that would explain how sick I knew she was.

NEVER GIVE UP ON SOMETHING THAT YOU CAN'T GO A DAY WITHOUT THINKING ABOUT —WINSTON CHURCHILL

I knew I needed to find another naturopath for her. It was eating me up. Even though I did what I was taught, it just wasn't enough. I found 11 naturopaths in the area in the phone book and then I found myself on another mission. I had no idea how hard this was going to be. For the next few months I made appointments and one by one I took her to see every one of them. Most of them were not hands-on; they didn't work on the cranium. Mostly they did herbal medications. I did learn something from all of them—I learned about different vitamins and minerals and what their role was to keep the body healthy. I always felt better when I was doing something to better my knowledge of the human body. Everything I learnt I felt I was one step closer to figuring out what she needed.

It was very interesting that while on this path of knowledge the genetics doctor called and asked my permission for a team of genetics doctors in the US to have Trina as their main case study for research on her very rare 3p minus syndrome. I was ecstatic. Finally, maybe there would be some answers for us. After talking with them and learning more about what it was they were trying to figure out from their research, my heart sank when I was told this would probably never help Trina. The studies took years and they still felt that Trina didn't have a lot of years. She was still in the same category as the other children even though she didn't have the same problems with her organs that the other children had. Anyway, I agreed to help. I was never selfish that way. I always wished well for others. They also asked me if they could put my name and number on a list for other parents around the world with rare syndromes. This would allow them to contact me and talk about what they were going through and because of our similar children maybe we could help each other. I also agreed to this. I felt that the more people there were to talk with, the better. The doctor that called explained to me more about the research. They were trying to find what genes were in the piece of the third chromosome that these children

Denise F. Loewen

were missing. If they could find out, they may be able to give the children what they were lacking. This was a very huge step as at this time researchers didn't know a lot about the genes that created the body. There were steps to take; first we would have to send our blood to the US—mine, her father's, and Trina's. This was not as easy as it sounds; everything had to be prearranged by the hospitals to have our blood sent. This process had to be done more than once. Either the live blood cells died before they arrived, or it would be stopped at the border for reasons I didn't know about. It took a few times, but we did finally succeed. Once that procedure was accomplished communication kind of ended there.

It was exciting and proud thinking that my Trina could help other children in the future; they had picked her not just because the syndrome was rare but also because she was so advanced. But I needed to stay focused on what I could do to help my daughter in the present. I continued to search for another naturopath, but none of them could help her. When they met with her they were honest and didn't string me along and try to get me to do things just to make money. I was definitely a walking target for that. I was very grateful that they didn't take advantage of us. This didn't help me find someone that could do for her what her first naturopath did. My next step was going to massage therapists. I thought maybe they would have some experience with cranial therapy. It was heart-wrenching at times—many of them tried to do a session with her. I did not blame them for not feeling comfortable with her. By this time Trina did not like to be touched. She screamed a lot and this was too much for them. We went to all of them, with no luck. Then it was chiropractors. I did find one that was able to do treatments on her. He was very gentle and she did respond to him. She liked to go so I knew it helped, but she needed more. There was one more therapist to take Trina to, the last one that I could find. I almost didn't make an appointment for her; I was so discouraged and felt that it was hard on Trina. Because I was desperate, I took her anyway.

This part of Trina's life deserves a whole book of its own. This appointment gave me hope and knowledge that would change both of us. The day of the appointment Trina was having a very bad day. She'd had a few seizures the night before and when she woke up I could tell just getting to the appointment was going to be a challenge. I found the address; once inside the building I stood at the bottom of a lot of stairs. I took a deep breath, looked at Trina and said come on baby we can do this. She was yelling and did not want to go up the steps. One step at a time, a few people were coming down the stairs or going up. They just looked at us but didn't say anything. I apologized for Trina's yelling and kept on. We made it. We were at the top. I had little hope that this was going to work anyway and felt bad for putting her through this. I had noticed she was possibly getting a phobia, or something. She was never afraid to go anywhere and now it seemed like she was afraid of smaller spaces, such as elevators or public washrooms. I couldn't put my finger on it, but things were definitely getting worse. All my attention was on trying to calm Trina down; I sang to her, I tried to rub her back. She was having none of it.

Once in the room, I introduced Trina and myself. We tried to get Trina to get on the massage table so she could do an assessment on her. It didn't work. Trina threw herself on the floor and I couldn't coax her to get up. I knew it was over before it even started. Now I was worried about how I was going to get her back down those steps. I tried explaining that

Denise F. Loewen

Trina had headaches and seizures. She asked me a little bit about Trina, whether Trina understood what we were saying and trying to do. I told her at this point I didn't think Trina was aware of anything. We did this all while she lay on the floor yelling. I knew there were other businesses in the building and felt bad, but there was nothing I could do but wait her out and hope she calmed down.

The next thing I knew, the therapist was on the floor with Trina, talking softly to her. She cupped Trina's head in her hands and just held her head. I didn't say a word; I just watched and backed off a little. She was the first one who didn't seem scared to touch Trina. After a while Trina calmed down and stopped screaming and I watched her little body completely relax. She laid on the floor with this beautiful lady holding her head and talking kindly to her. I froze; I'm sure I stopped breathing for a bit. Trina fell asleep right there on the floor. We talked about what Trina was going through. I was very honest about how I felt with her diagnosis. I didn't agree that her syndrome had anything to do with her behavior, and that's why I was there. I also told her I understood if she couldn't work with Trina because of the yelling when we first got there. She agreed it would be hard, and she needed to be respectful of the other people in the building. I couldn't believe it when she suggested she come to our house and work on Trina. She felt Trina would feel more comfortable in her own home. She looked at Trina and we both agreed that what she did for her in those few minutes was the most relief she had had in a long time. We let her sleep while we talked. This wonderful woman told me a little about herself and that she had worked on children with autism and had had very good results. This treatment was called Ortho-Bionomy, light touch healing. I had never heard of this before, but it sounded very interesting. What I liked about it most was that it didn't cause any pain or discomfort for Trina while she was having the treatment done. It wasn't the same as her naturopath did; it was working with the muscles not the bones. We agreed that once a week on Fridays around 8:30 pm. would be a good time. Trina would be sleeping then.

This was the start of a new beginning for not just Trina but for my other children and for myself. I was and am forever grateful for the miracle that took place in that little room way up those stairs. I started a new journey of learning and Trina was relieved from pain and serious problems that she would have faced in the future. I looked forward to Fridays. Trina never woke up while having her treatment and she was always more relaxed for the next few days afterward. I would watch while the treatment was happening and after a few weeks I started to ask questions. I was amazed at how she responded. One evening while Trina was getting her treatment, I was asking questions about how she knew what Trina's body was doing, and how did she know what she needed to do. This was the evening when I learned hands-on how to read Trina's body energy. It was incredible. The energy flow of the muscles in someone else's body was amazing. The fact that I could tune into her flow and feel her muscles moving under my fingers, well I don't have the right words. All I know is that after that evening with the help of her therapist, and with what I had learned from her naturopath, I myself was on a whole new path of being able to help my daughter. I started to take classes on Ortho-Bionomy. I had the best teacher—she knew why I wanted to learn how to do this amazing treatment. I was able to work with Trina almost right away. The incredible thing about this whole thing was that I was now able to help her every day so she didn't have to wait until Fridays.

Denise F. Loewen

WHEN ONE DOOR CLOSES
ANOTHER ONE OPENS

I felt like I was doing something to help Trina—feeling helpless is so hard when you know there's something hurting your child. The treatments were relieving some of her pain and she seized less. I knew this was something that Trina benefited from as she would often place my hands on her head and want a treatment done. She did not want to be touched or hugged much now, so this was definitely helping her. I knew I needed to keep on learning and trying to figure out what was making her sick. Her body didn't look healthy— she was all puffy. She was hurting and I couldn't pinpoint it.

Trina was having a hard time being away from me. She still loved going to school and her TA was very good with her. When at school she would ask for me all day long. Her schedule board showed her what her day was going to look like. At the end of the day she could put "Mom" up on her board. Her teacher said when they couldn't get her to focus on any of her other tasks and she kept putting Mom up on the board that's how they knew she needed me. Everyone knew that if Trina needed me they only had to call and I would come and get her. I never felt she should be at school if she couldn't handle it.

A huge change became more apparent during the ages of 13 to 15. Trina had started to show signs of phobias, but they became extreme. It was hard enough to take her out shopping or just on a regular outing with the other kids, but now she was terrified of public washrooms, elevators, and even going into buildings other than our house or her school. As a family I think we were amazing—all of my kids were so gentle with her and totally understood if we had to make a shopping trip short or had to cancel.

These phobias became so bad that we would have to go all the way home if Trina had to pee. She would drop to the floor if I tried to make her go into a small space. This was not Trina at all; she had loved to ride elevators and always felt comfortable using any washroom. She loved to go out shopping and go on drives. Going out and doing family things was never an issue with Trina, so when these behaviors got so bad it stopped us from doing things that needed to be done, I knew Trina was getting sicker and sicker.

She also started to have hallucinations during seizures. At first I thought (and maybe I was right, but couldn't prove it) that her hallucinations made her scared of the things she loved to do. When she would come out of a seizure there were times when she was scared of me and would try to run away from me. This was very difficult because I couldn't let her go after a seizure. Her balance was extremely bad and she would fall. It broke my heart to think that she was seeing something that was not there and couldn't tell me what she saw. This made it very hard for her to function at school if her class was going out on outing. Her new TA did not understand that Trina was sick. Her aggressive behavior toward her new teacher was taken personally. She tried to tell me that Trina was lashing out on purpose and was a danger to society. This is when I took her out of the school system. It was hard enough trying to get doctors to listen to me and not think I was crazy for thinking she was sick. I didn't need a TA who was with my daughter every day turning against her and making her out as though she was intentionally trying to hurt people.

Denise F. Loewen

I knew Trina was in pain, but even I didn't know how much. Trina had half of a school year left in elementary school. I tried to get a different TA for my daughter but the school system would not back me. I knew the two did not fit together and because Trina was non-verbal I felt her safety was at risk. I kept her home for the rest of the year. This was hard on her; she loved school, but I knew she was getting worse and could not tolerate being with someone who didn't understand her. I needed to be the one with her all the time.

Some days all I wanted to do was hold her and rock her. I read anything I could think of. I was now a single parent and at times I felt very alone. Those feelings never lasted long; I had the best kids in the world. They loved their sister and wanted for her to be healthy as much as I did. They remembered how happy and loving she was before she got sick. They protected her from the cruel words from outsiders as much as they could. I knew in my heart that if they could be this strong and always be at her side, I could be stronger and never give up the fight to get someone to listen to me. At this time I had people in the professional field telling me Trina would be better off in a group home. There she would get the services that I could not get for her because she was my natural child. This did not make any sense to me. I worked for the system and knew what was available, but in a group home she would not have had me, and I was the most important person in her life. I knew that without me her life would not only be shortened, but it would be a life of drugs to sedate her and keep her calm. That would have killed her; her actions were her voice. Without being able to act, she would not be heard. Until I had more people in my life who believed that she was sick, I choose to take care of her myself.

I was seeing a pattern to the changes that were happening to her. What I saw was every time she had a good growth spurt, her medication would be increased. With each increase her anger would get worse. I didn't know if this could be an answer, but I wasn't going to rule anything out. It was important to me to look at every change in her life and how it affected her. When talking to her doctors about this, they did not agree with me.

So, once again, I started to research. I looked into the clobazam seizure medication that she was on. When she was put on this medication I was told there were very few side effects. I took this to be true. She had been on this medication for six years now. To me it didn't make any sense to not try and take her off it. Her health was poor and she had no joy in life. I knew the older she became the more difficult it would be to have her in school and to take her in social settings. The other problem with her age was that she was getting closer to the age that all the other children with her syndrome lived to be. This was brought up to me more times than I can remember. When I would take her to the hospital and she was seen by specialists, that is what they told me they had read when learning about her syndrome. I knew they were wrong; it wasn't her syndrome that was keeping her from being healthy, but I also knew I could not convince the doctors of this.

It didn't take me long to discover that one of the side effects from the seizure medication was extreme violent outbursts. The very idea that this could happen to my daughter was unthinkable. The first thing I did was to take her to our family doctor and let him know what I had found. I really don't think he felt that this was the problem, but he did listen to me. Trina was still having seizures, and they were getting

Denise F. Loewen

worse. We couldn't keep increasing her medication—it was time for us to give her body a break. I wanted her off the drug, as I was sure this was adding to her anger. We slowly reduced the seizure medication. Her seizures didn't get worse, but her screaming, anger, and phobias didn't get better either.

It was a tough decision to make and I didn't have any of the doctors on my side, this I knew. I wanted her off the medication even though things didn't change. I made this decision because her seizures didn't get worse so I saw no reason for her to be on them. I did get the okay from our family doctor and that's all I needed. Even though I was on my own I felt better about what I had done—I could concentrate on the now and not wonder if her difficulties were medication induced.

When I remember her days of life back then, oh how I wish I could do it over again, knowing then what I know now. I tried my best to keep her out of the hospital and away from other doctors. They had no positive information for me; it was always the same thing. She has a very rare syndrome and her assessment from the genetics team that said she had a behavior problem was the only thing that they seemed to focus on. That and the fact that they thought I wanted them to make her normal, which was the furthest thing from my mind. My daughter was beautiful and she was one of the best things that had happen to me in my lifetime. She loved life, and people. She touched souls everywhere she went. I know it wasn't their fault, but the professionals just thought this was the way she was and there was nothing wrong with her medically—that she was mentally challenged and would not get any better ever and I just needed to accept this fact.

Every time I left the hospital or her specialists' appointments I would drive home talking to her all the way. Letting her know that it's okay Trina, I don't believe them and that's not how I feel. I will figure it out, I promise. I prayed, I cried, and I screamed with her. There were times when I would give it back to the Earth—when I was overwhelmed and was losing faith and energy I would give it back. I believed that God only gives to us what we can handle, but sometimes I thought he was expecting too much of me, and my little girl was paying the price.

YOU NEVER KNOW HOW STRONG YOU ARE
UNTIL BEING STRONG IS THE
ONLY CHOICE YOU HAVE
—CAYLA MILLS

Denise F. Loewen

My Inner Teacher Speaks Again

Please keep your mind open while reading this—I thought I was losing my mind after having this dream. Then I figured out what it meant and what I was supposed to learn from it. Sometimes letting God know that he has overwhelmed you is the right thing to do.

I'm in this huge kitchen and there are kids running around and laughing. (This is a life that is real to me; being a foster parent, this is how my kitchen was most of the time.) I'm making them some lunch. I am talking with the bigger children and the little ones are at my feet. I am feeling so happy and full of love. All my kids are there and many more, I don't even know how many. I'm asking them what they would like for lunch, all together they yell soup, soup; we all laughed. I tell them to go play so I can make them their soup. The older children take the little ones and away they go. Now it's quiet in the kitchen. All the children have left; I can hear them faintly in the background. I'm happy and content. I remember I'm standing at the counter with a can of soup in my hands. I pick up a can opener that was lying on the counter. I start opening the can, I'm not looking down. I've done this so many times I can do it with my eyes closed. Something doesn't feel right to me. I have a sick feeling in my stomach—so much that I'm afraid to look down at what I'm doing. I look and what I see makes me scream out loud. Trina is standing in front of me and I'm opening the top of her head with the can opener. My screaming wakes me up.

I feel sick, I'm crying and shaking. I've had nightmares before but never anything so gruesome that I can't shake it for days. I had so many feelings about this dream; first I thought I was going crazy. I talked to a close friend about it. I didn't want anyone to know that I felt I was losing it. I picked this friend to tell because she was very close to our family and I knew she would understand the stress I was under. Her wise words to me was to stop thinking I was going crazy and try and put it together with what was happening in my life.

Dreams teach us so much if we pay attention to them. My friend and I talked about Trina and how hopeless I was feeling. I just didn't think I was getting any closer to figuring out why she was so sick. I told her about all the changes Trina was going through and how she was getting worse. We talked about her syndrome and how I wished they had never diagnosed her with it. I showed her the letter that I received from her assessment and how angry I was about it. How it just made everything worse for us.

Talking this over with someone who didn't look down on me for fighting the system and not giving in helped me calm down and really look at the dream in a different way. I had been asking the doctors to please keep looking and doing tests that would explain what was happening to her. Thinking about the chromosome disorder and the enzymes that should be in the piece that's missing, I finally realized that the dream was telling me to feed her brain. When I was able to step back and really see what I was being shown, that's what I got out of the dream. I once again had something to learn and some hope that I could help her on my own.

Denise F. Loewen

So I start reading about vitamins and minerals—what they do for us and how they affect us when we are lacking in a certain one. There was so much to learn. I asked questions, many questions. I found a health drink that had all the nutrients in it to feed the body and brain. I read about the omega oils and how they can help the brain for children with ADHD and autism. I had Trina tested for autism when she was younger, mainly for services. With Trina being diagnosed with a rare syndrome that nobody had heard of she didn't fit in any category for services. They would not say that she was autistic because she was too aware of her surroundings. She was also very social with people. She didn't have autism, and yet she showed autistic tendencies as she got sicker. She was repetitive with her words; she did puzzles over and over again. She attached herself to playing cards. She sorted them and carried them with her all the time.

I knew I was on the right track. Trina started feeling a bit better. The first thing I noticed was that her seizures slowed down. This was after months mind you; she was back in school by then, and even her teachers noticed a difference. Things were starting to look a little better for her. It was a slow process, but every second of my time reading and meeting with people who could help was worth it. I found another naturopath who could help me with the nutritional part of her health. I tried to get help from the government to help pay for some of her vitamins. This was another fight that took time and energy away from my kids. I never thought that wanting her to have something that actually helped her feel better would be met with a "no." They would pay hundreds of dollars a month to keep her on a drug that was making her sick, but would not help with natural nutrition that was making her feel better. I took on this mission for months. Her teachers at her new school were willing to help me. They definitely saw a big improvement in her health and behaviour.

So I started to write letters and her teachers wrote letters on her behalf. I really thought I could make a difference, not only for Trina but also for other children who needed vitamins and minerals to help keep them healthy. I would get letters back but they always sent me to another department. Every time I'd have to do it all over again. This went on for almost a year, then I receive a letter from the government saying that they had reviewed my request and it was decided that even though Trina was feeling better they could not change the system for one child. That was that. I knew I didn't have the strength or the time to fight them any longer.

I gave up asking for help and started working harder. I had to do it on my own, that I knew for sure. I think I would have continued with my request if I hadn't found the means to buy what she needed myself. The strength would have come from somewhere, that I am sure of. When you have a child who depends on you for everything, some kind of energy grows inside of you that you have no idea where it comes from. Every day you surprise yourself. I knew that as long as Trina had fight left in her, I was sure I could match it.

I'll be honest with you, though—there were days when I doubted myself. I didn't know where I would get the energy to get up in the morning. That is, if I had gotten any sleep at all during the night. I went to Trina every time she had a seizure and that sometimes kept me awake most of the night. Most of my doubt would be after a doctor's appointment or a stay at the hospital. It never lasted long. A smile or a hug from Trina would get me right back on track. She was such a courageous child to come to this Earth to teach others what she had to teach. She taught our family something new every day. Patience, kindness, and forgiveness are a few things that come to mind. I found a quote that reminds me of Trina and the powerful energy that she shared with all those who cared to listen and learn. Even though she couldn't say this in words, she sure said it loudly with her actions.

COURAGE IS LOOKING FEAR IN THE
EYES AND SAYING, GET THE HELL OUT
OF MY WAY, I'VE GOT THINGS TO DO

We moved into a different house. It was perfect for us. It had lots of bedrooms and space to play. The best thing about it was it had a swimming pool and a huge yard. Trina loved to be outside—this was so good for her.

Trina had a hard time in the community because of her phobias, which I still couldn't get a handle on. Things didn't change drastically, but rather, slowly. I was taking her to a naturopath; she was still getting her Ortho-Bionomy treatments. I also found a chiropractor that she really liked. He was gentle and was not afraid of her loud yelling or fear of being touched. Another therapy that I discovered was Brain Gym. It was very helpful for Trina's fears. It was something that fit for her and she enjoyed. She would do her brain therapy on her own when she was printing or doing her puzzles. Every one of these therapies helped her in different ways. Her teachers at school were always open to learning new things that helped Trina progress. I never turned down any information that might help. Learning made me feel like I was getting closer to an answer.

I loved my daughter and never forgot how kind and gentle she was before she got sick and I always showed her gentleness and kindness. The angrier she got the gentler I got. I never gave up showing her gentle touches and kind voices. We all sang to her and sat with her. She was never left alone when she had a seizure, even though some of the doctors told me that what I was doing with her while she seized was not helping bring her out of them. I never got sucked into that message that I was wasting my time by being there whenever she needed me. I began to feel that they were more worried about my health than hers. This just made me angry with them. I could take care of myself and knew when I needed help. I wanted them to hear my words and stop telling me there was nothing that they could do for Trina. I stopped taking her to the big city hospitals after they wrote the letter that changed any positive opinion that her future doctors would have as far as listening to me went. Maybe that was wrong of me and maybe not. They were honest about not knowing any more than I did about my daughter. Actually, they knew less than I did.

Day after day things got worse for her. The school year ended so I didn't have to worry about elementary school any longer. Once high school started for her she would have a new TA. I couldn't believe she was going to be in high school— the time went by so fast. Her health was not improving fast enough to keep up with the illness that I knew was destroying her inside. Her eating habits had changed long ago, but now all she wanted to eat was eggs. Eggs for every meal. She wanted them so bad that she would go into the fridge and get the eggs out. I can't count how many eggs got broke during this time. I could not see what was going on but I could tell by how she acted and how her body showed signs of being very ill. The swelling of her body continued to worsen. She slept less and less—it was getting so that she was crash sleeping.

Denise F. Loewen

She would go hard with physical activities. The yelling and the hallucinations while she seized was like something out of the movies. I was sick for her; I would call our family doctor and try to explain to him what was happening to her. He could hear her screaming right beside me, and then he asked me if I wanted an ambulance to come and put her in the mental ward at the hospital. I didn't know what to do for her. I did know what I didn't want to do to her. She wasn't crazy. She was sick. I thanked him for his time and told him I would figure out something to do for her. I know he had no idea either; he wanted for us both to be safe.

This one episode sticks in my head and I'll never forget that feeling of "fight or flight." Trina had fallen asleep and she had a very scary seizure; she was hallucinating and something in her hallucination was around her on her bed. She was trying to catch whatever it was in the air. All of a sudden, she caught whatever it was. It scared her so much that she started screaming and trying to climb the wall. I was talking to her and keeping her safe, but she was so scared she wouldn't let me touch her. When she came out of it, she wanted to go outside; I let her go and went with her. She ended up at the school down the street. She started running on the track and ran for so long, like she was running away some something. She ran until she was exhausted. She lay on the ground and I lay down beside her. Together we looked up in the sky, I didn't say anything to her—we were both silent. Trina finally looked at me and quietly said, "Home." I took her by the hand and together we walked home. I got her ready for bed and she went to sleep.

There were more and more of these days. I would take her to our family doctor and try and explain things to him and make him believe me. I know in my heart he wanted to, but he just could never find any medical problem to work with. When I look back at those days now I really can't believe he stuck with us all those years. Sometimes when we'd go to see him, Trina would be yelling and couldn't sit in the waiting room. I would walk her up and down the hallway for however long it took to get in to see him. I did my best to keep her quiet as to not disturb the other patients. I'm sure some of them complained, but most, I believe, where very understanding and felt sorry for Trina, maybe for both of us. I would get questions like, "Does she live at home with you?" When I would tell them yes their would response would be how brave I was and usually everyone would wish us luck. Most people were very kind.

I will be forever grateful to our family doctor for not giving up on us, even when I'm sure many times he wished we would just go away. He was more than a doctor to us; he would listen and spend time getting to know Trina. It was for me being her mom and not able to help her and I'm sure he felt the same being her doctor and not having any answers for us.

I spent one morning recently watching videos of Trina during this time of her life. I have a hard time watching them. So many feelings rush over me. She was so wonderful. The videos were taken at school. She was playing basketball and catch with her TA in the big gym. She was so good at shooting baskets and dribbling the ball. Her keen eye and quick responses still shows me that she would have been able to enjoy life and would have accomplished so much more had she not been sick. Another video was her reading her sight words, she loved reading and writing. There was one of Trina at gymnastics club jumping on the trampoline with the biggest smile ever on her face. I watched her playing ball with the other kids. She was so proud of herself when she did

Denise F. Loewen

her seat drops and would get right back on her feet without missing a beat. Listening to her laugh and talking, well what can I say; it puts a smile on my face. She may have been special needs, but she had beat the one thing that should have taken her as an infant—3p minus syndrome. It's hard to believe she could still function through all of the pain and seizures during this time. Watching her with her TA gives me a whole new feeling of gratitude. Sometimes I would forget just how great her teachers were to her. I am and will forever be grateful for them, and I know that Trina loves them still. She showed how much she cared for them; when she would have a new teacher in her life it took her a long time to let go of the one that worked with her before. She would ask for them by name over and over.

Her poor little body was so puffy; you could tell the discomfort she was in by the way she walked and bent down. She had slowed down so much from the two years before. I'm so glad now that I could be there for her every hour of the day.

I just couldn't believe that she was saved twice already from death and this was how she was suppose to live. No way. I wouldn't accept it. I would do anything I had to do to get someone anyone to listen to me. I found someone who did reflexology. I had talked to many people and I had been told that working on the feet could help with many problems. This wonderful lady came to our home and tried to do a treatment on Trina. When she left she said she was sorry but she just couldn't work on her. She felt Trina was in too much pain to handle it.

I was on a mission; I talked to whoever would listen to me. Friends, family, teachers, even people from health food stores. I shared her story and told it so many times I felt like our lives were a skipping record. I was so worried about her health that sometimes I forgot that she was still progressing with school. I had to grow with her and do things that challenged her mind and learn new techniques to stimulate her brain. I knew I had to keep her brain learning—this was important to me because when she was better she would not have lost all the knowledge that she had worked so hard to learn. She loved music and was learning how to use the computers. She loved to watch shows on TV like Jeopardy and other shows of knowledge. Her favorite was The Price Is Right. She couldn't tell time, but knew always what time it was. She knew when her shows were on and she would stop whatever she was doing at that time and come running into the house, turn on her TV and sit down to watch her show. Using the remote, she could watch more than one show at a time. She was so smart. As long as she had any kind of fight in her I was not going to stop fighting for her. I never forgot about the doctor that told me to never let anyone tell me she wasn't smart.

Unfortunately, she ended up in the hospital with seizures again. The neurologist that came to the hospital had another medication that we had not tried yet. I felt like I was dammed if I did and dammed if I didn't. I had this fear inside me that if I didn't put her on these medications that the doctors wanted to try and I lost her I would be the cause of her death. The fear ran stronger that my gut feeling that the medication was going to make her sicker. Always her body had shown us that if there was a side effect from any medication, even if only a one percent chance, it was going to happen. The hardest part about putting her on new medications was that she couldn't tell you verbally what was happening inside of her. I would have to wait until the signs were visual and then beg for the

Denise F. Loewen

doctors to listen to me. Doing this to her set her back in every way. She would stop talking and miss school; she would lose days or weeks of her life while her body fought the side effects of these drugs. I never really knew the depth of what the side effects did to her, only what I could see.

Within hours of me giving Trina the new seizure medication the side effects started. The school was aware that she was on a new drug. (Topamax this time.) She was only at school for a few hours when the school phoned and told me Trina was having some serious side effects from this new drug. It took three people to get her home. They decided to record her on video so I could show her doctors what happened to her. I was so grateful that they understood and did everything they could to help her. They knew how hard it was for me to explain what she was going through; taking her to the hospital didn't work for that. It felt like they just thought she was always like that, aggressive and had a behavior problem. I even tried to take her to the hospital when she wasn't sick so they could see that she was loving or and could walk on her own. That didn't really help as the staff changed so much and I couldn't take her into ER if she wasn't sick.

The video did help. I took it to her neurologist the next day asked him to watch it so he could see this was not the right thing to do to her; he agreed she should come of immediately. I know to a doctor that works with the brain it didn't make sense to him to not have her on medication. I got that, but I also knew she was sick and if they could figure out what it was that was making her so sick maybe her seizures would go away on their own. I felt if it was just epilepsy then why had the medications not work. It would have made me feel a little better if there was even one answer that made sense to my questions. I would not, could not accept her syndrome as the answer to everything that was wrong. I had to be careful not to let up and to be in the medicals field's eyes enough so they wouldn't just forget about her, but not so much that they would think I was crazy and maybe have her taken from me. Might seem like I was being paranoid, but that was a legitimate worry that most parents with special needs children have thought about. I needed the professionals in the medical field to respect that I knew my child better than anyone else on the planet. I did respect them for their knowledge of the medical field, and I just wanted the same in return.

Denise F. Loewen

Never Give Up—Your Victory Could Be Right Around the Corner

As I have said, I was committed to fighting alongside Trina as long as she had any fight in her. Well, Trina stopped fighting. She became so ill that she began to lose her ability to function. She seized more and more. At first she stopped walking, and then she stopped eating on her own. She was too sick to go to school so I started to keep her home with me. For months I fed her I had to put Pull-Ups on her. She didn't understand why she had to wear them. We spent hours and hours in the bathroom. She would ask to go pee over and over; she would sit on the toilet and nothing. She wanted to go but couldn't. Her bladder would release on her without her being able to control it. I didn't know a lot about this problem—it was a new one for me. Now once again I had something new I had to learn about. I needed to understand how the bladder worked. She'd had a few urinary infections over the last years; this I learned was from her bladder not being able to empty properly or could be from constipation. She ended up having a few surgeries to open her urinary tract. This happens because after repeated infections scar tissue builds up and needs to be removed surgically. After each surgery she would be fine again—she could pee and she would be good for about a year. I knew what to look for when this was happening, but now there was no infection she had had the surgery done and still she couldn't pee.

Now another fear was with me—all of the other children with 3p minus had passed away from kidney failure. Trina had not had problems with her kidneys and bladder like the other children. Our family doctor did test after test for me, checking everything he could think of to find a cause for this. Every test he did came back normal. Trina was above average in heath with every test possible. There was no explanation. How was it possible that a child who was so extremely healthy was losing all normal functions? I couldn't wrap my head around this. She would end up in the hospital, they would do the same tests over each time we were there, and nothing was found. They would stop her seizures with Valium; it didn't take much I guess because she wasn't on anything else. Soon they gave me a prescription for Valium so I could give it to her at home; there was nothing they could do for her anyway. They would let her sleep and ask me if I wanted to leave her there. I always refused, I knew they were trying to help but I knew if I let them have her she would not live long. I was always very thankful, and let them know how much I appreciated their help. I always took her home with me. This is how her life was now every day. I was lost and scared I didn't have anyone else to turn to. There was no answer for her being so ill.

I spent every day taking care of her. I fed her and changed her. I made sure she got up to walk around. She was losing interest in the things she enjoyed doing—her puzzles became very difficult and she stopped reading and writing. She didn't want to swim any more. She was afraid of the water. Some days she didn't want to have a bath. This was very unusual

Denise F. Loewen

for her as she loved the water. It had always been the one thing that would calm her down and make her feel relaxed. Friends would come and check on us.

Everyone was very worried about her. They would listen to me and give me the courage and the strength to keep fighting for her. Jackie, who had grown up and moved away from home, came back. She needed to be with her little sister as much as we needed her back to help. Jonathon was living in town. He would take his sister for overnight visits—my God when I think of how wonderful he was with his sister! He did this to give me a break and to spend time with her. Trina just couldn't get enough of them. My older foster children helped, too. I never felt like I was alone, just desperate.

I still went to our family doctor, but there were many appointments where Trina was too sick to go. I would talk to him and tell him the problems that I was dealing with. Some days were better than others, but there were fewer good days and more sick days. He would listen and sometimes get me to have some blood work done, and some days he didn't know what to say. He always made me feel like he cared. I know in my heart when he would tell me he thought about her and would try to help me find an answer that he meant it. I remember getting very emotional during this time. I was never a crier, I learned early in life that didn't really solve things. Many times people would say things like, "It must be so hard. You should take a holiday and take some time for yourself," or, "I couldn't do what you do with her." They said this because they cared about me. I felt then and still feel now that I don't regret one minute of my life with her. She needed me to keep her safe from what could happen to her should she end up in the hospital without me. The thought made me sick to my stomach. Because Trina was non-verbal and did not understand what was being done to her when we were there, without me they would have strapped her down and drugged her up. This I know for a fact. They would feel this was keeping her safe and no one but me was going to stay at her side the whole time she was in the hospital. I understand it in my brain, but not in my heart. Having that done to her would surely have made her lose her mind. She was not one to give up easily. When people would say they couldn't do it, well maybe not, but if it was their child I'm sure they would give it all they had. We use to say to Trina when she would go for days sometimes without sleeping, "You sure picked the right family, Trina." But there was nothing we wouldn't do for her.

It doesn't seem possible that she could get even sicker and not have anything wrong with her that the doctors could find. I don't even know what kept me going every day and to keep her alive. I just don't know and can't find words to describe it. Her days were lying on the couch, being fed, and wearing diapers. The doctors blamed this on her syndrome. She was close to 17 years old. None of the other 3p minus children lived to be adults. While this seemed to be the easiest explanation for the doctors, every cell of my being did not agree. If that's what it was then why was her heart so strong, and why did she have no kidney problems? All her blood work said that she was above average in health with every test they did. And yet she was failing. I was losing her right before my eyes and there was not a damn thing I could do about it except keep talking, stay in contact with the one doctor who wanted to help and gave up on her. (If he did he didn't show me.)

I honestly don't remember some of those days, but I do remember taking her to our family doctor again. This could have been the last time she was that sick. I begged him to do

Denise F. Loewen

the test again but he called me on it this time. He said that they had done them they showed nothing.

"Please just one more time," I pleaded. "Maybe we missed something; we can't just give up on her." We talked about her syndrome again and I don't remember what I said, but he agreed. One more time. Oh, my God, as sick as she was I managed to get her to the clinic for her blood work. I basically had to carry her in there. The girls at the lab were so nice to us; they knew Trina very well and always talked to her with kindness. They let me know it will take a few days to get the blood work results back. They always wished us luck and gave me a smile.

I felt good; I don't know why, realistically the test results would show nothing wrong like every other time. Maybe because even getting that done I felt like I was doing something for her. She wasn't eating much anymore and had a hard time using her hands. She had stopped talking; she would just repeat "Mom, Mom, Mom" over and over again. All I could do was hold her and promise her I would figure it out. "I promise," I told her.

She mostly slept and seized. She wasn't yelling or fussing anymore. It kind of reminded me of how she was before they had done her stomach surgery for pyloric stenosis when she was six months old. I was losing her again and didn't know why. When I would massage her and rub her back or do the Ortho-Bionomy treatments for her, she didn't respond much. Not like she use to. I slept beside her and talked her through every seizure. I really didn't care if they thought it helped or not. I knew it did.

I was scared, that's a fact. I was scared to have her at home, but I was more scared to have her in the hospital. It might sound crazy, but I didn't feel she would be safe there.

At least no one was trying to talk me into doing something I didn't want to do with her. I was not strong enough at this point to not lose it on them. Everyone has a breaking point. I knew mine and it was best to stay away from those who didn't have faith in her and felt that her life was over.

Over those few days, Trina was not getting any better. I was doing everything in my power to keep her with us. I fed her soft foods and gave her liquids with an eyedropper. I needed to keep her hydrated so she wouldn't end up in the hospital. I knew that if her health got any worse we would be there anyway. She was so swollen and puffy; her seizures were full grand mal seizures now. She was getting tired, that I could tell; she had very little strength left. We all cried while taking care of her; everyone was so gentle with her and so helpful for me.

Then it happened—the phone rang and it was her doctor. He asked me to come to the office. Trina's blood work was back. I managed to have someone watch her and I drove downtown. I was not thinking good thoughts: "Why does he need to see me? What did he find that he didn't find before? There must be something or he would have waited until our next appointment." So many things were going through my mind. I wanted to get there as fast as I could and yet I was scared to hear what he had to say. Whatever it was, it would be better than not knowing. (Even while writing this, my heart beat so fast and my brain was thinking faster than I could type.)

I sat in the waiting room and he came in with a paper in his hand. I knew this was her test results. He told me they found something, but first he wants to go over all the tests results with me. There are two pages of results. He slowly shows me each one. They all read average and above average.

Denise F. Loewen

I don't understand. Everything about her is above average. Her organs are all working great, her blood levels are at the best they can be. This is all the same as every other test we had done. Except one thing. He pointed to the bottom of the page and in his own handwriting was written "vitamin B12." Her level was so low that it was hardly readable. It was a miracle that she was still alive.

I couldn't breathe. It was true: there was something wrong and she would get better. I was shaking, he wanted me to go home and bring her to the office so he could give her her first shot. I can't tell you how I got her there, but I did. I sat with her while he gave her a double shot of vitamin B12. That's what was making her so sick. You can't live without it. It's what keeps your brain healthy and communicating with the rest of your body. On the way home I stopped to tell Jackie what had just happened. Another miracle—my son was at his sister's when I arrived there. That in itself was a sign that we were all meant to be together. We cried and hugged and thanked God for not taking Trina. When I told my brother, Trina's uncle he couldn't even speak. He would ask me the same questions over and over again. He just couldn't believe that all those years he watched his niece suffer, for what? He never got over the anger that he felt. His love for Trina showed every time he saw her when he hugged her tight. Within 48 hours of getting her first shot she was up and walking. I will be forever grateful to our doctor for not giving up on her and having faith in me. He wanted me to bring her in once a week for a shot until her levels were up to normal. It wasn't happening like that. Once Trina realized that it was the shot that was making her feel better, she started to ask for the doctor and wanted to go see him. We went every three days from then on. There were tears of joy now when we went to the office; she would look in his hand to see if he had the needle for her, then he got a huge hug. She was a miracle. That's a fact. She was here for a reason and her teachings here on this Earth were not done yet.

Remember my dream about opening the can of soup and it was the top of Trina's head? That dream kept her alive when she should have gone back to Heaven. There was only one explanation how she survived being so deficient of vitamin B12. I started to give her extra vitamins and minerals as soon as I figured what that dream had meant to me. The research that I had done on what the body needs to stay healthy was what saved her. I learned about vitamin B12 and had been giving her B complex along with many other vitamins and minerals. When I was able to talk with her doctor more about how she could have been deficient when I was giving her B12. He explained that her tracking cells in her body had died when she was a baby. Because she was so sick from birth and was malnourished till she was six months old, this killed off her tracking cells. These are the cells that take the vitamin B12 from the bloodstream and carry it to the rest of the body. Without these cells her body couldn't take the B12 where it needed to go and it was not absorbed. I could have been giving her bowls of it every day and her body would not have received it. The only way to get it to her organs was to give her a shot. It's kind of like being a diabetic; she would need the B12 shots for the rest of her life. The horrible thing about all of this is that she suffered from this from about the age of six. When you're born your body has enough vitamin B12 stored in your organs from your mother that will last for about 5 years. Trina started to get aggressive at around the age of six. Remember she was very tiny and didn't start to grow until she was six or seven years old. This should have

Denise F. Loewen

been one of the first things that she was tested for when she had all the assessments done by the genetics team. All her information was given to them from me when we first started to see them. They knew how sick she was at birth and that she did not have surgery until she was six months old. They also knew she was diagnosed with failure to thrive when the pediatrician had discovered that she had pyloric stenosis. My research taught me that this was not a rare problem with malnutrition but a common one. Our family doctor never thought to check her B12 level; we had spent so much time with genetics it was assumed that they had already done it.

All those years of her life when she should have been playing and growing, and becoming the wonderful kid she was meant to be had been taken from her. She could have had a life without pain but instead she had horrible pain and no voice to express it to anyone. Her pain went away almost immediately; she never again had aggressive behavior, as they called it. The swelling of her body was all gone within a month of getting her first shot. She looked and felt like a different child. The puffiness on her forehead went away and so did her migraine headaches. She was coming back, and very quickly. And this is when I started to learn true forgiveness.

It only took weeks and she was back in school again. She was doing so much better that she now could be in a life skills program. This was a program that she couldn't attend because of her yelling, and once again I'll say it, "behavior." That word puts a knot in my stomach to this day and I'm sure will for the rest of my life. Forgiveness—that didn't come right away. I was so grateful to have my daughter back, laughing and jumping on the trampoline. She was talking again and enjoying the things in life that made her smile. My faith kept me strong, and watching her made everything worthwhile.

My anger only surfaced when I was alone. I wanted to hurt someone for making my little girl live in so much pain it almost killed her. From the age of six to seventeen, it's almost unthinkable that she suffered from a simple problem like a vitamin deficiency when so many specialists were on her case. The best they could do was blame me for not disciplining her enough. Instead of treating her like an individual, they typecast her into a group with ten other children; it was easier for them to place her in a category where she obviously did not belong—even I could see that. It just seemed that once she was diagnosed with a syndrome that was so rare it was easier for them to put the blame of their lack of knowledge on a little girl who was just sick. Their letter stating that she had a behavior problem when she was six followed her all those years. Was I angry? Yes. Am I angry? Yes, I am. But I also had my baby back and her brother and sister had their baby sister back. That's what we focused on—the positive. Trina wasn't angry. She was happy to be at school and do all the things that she loved. That's what she taught us. I was more grateful than angry. I couldn't change what happened, but I did learn from it. It made me stronger, and a better advocate for her. I was so proud of her and impressed with how fast she recovered. She was so beautiful and had so much more to teach. As to what we would learn from her, it was up to each and every one of us who had the privilege of being part of her life journey to realize.

Denise F. Loewen

Making Sense of it All

I was a mom. I was Trina's mom. I had three beautiful children and had no knowledge of illness or special needs until I had my daughter Trina. People who would run into me in the community would look at me as if they knew me. They would say to me, "You're the mom of the little girl with the long blonde hair?" Or, "You're Trina's mom?" I always smiled a proud smile; it seemed like anyone who met her never forgot her face or what a positive energy they felt when they were around her. This was amazing since most of these people knew Trina when she was screaming and fighting the pain that was inside her that no one could visually see. I'm sure for a while I had lost my own name and became "Trina's mom." That was a fit for me and never did I feel lost or non-existent in our world. I was so connected with her I would at times feel her pain.

During the time that she was so sick with the vitamin B12 deficiency I searched for spiritual guidance. Many a time throughout her life I would lose faith in my beliefs of a higher power. I remember that even at the times of my deepest anger at the universe, it was my higher power that I would talk to, ask questions of, and, yes, even yell and get angry at for the horrendous pain my daughter had to suffer. The more I learned about the deficiency the tighter my gut would become. I didn't get it.

Trina was loving and gentle again. We would sit together and do puzzles and laugh. She would hug us so tight as if she never wanted to let go. There was no more hitting and pushing me away. Her phobias stopped, she once again could go into any space in public buildings, and she could ride the elevator without dropping to her knees. Her eating habits went back to normal, she would eat foods with flavor and even though she still liked eggs, she stopped asking for them all the time. When I think about the eggs I think how smart she was and how she knew her own body. Eggs are a natural source of vitamin B12. If I only had put it together myself.

Watching her come back eased the pain in my heart and the feeling that I had failed her all those years. She showed me how to move on and love life for what it was. The more I understood the spiritual being that she was, the calmer and more forgiving I became. Instead of being angry I became a channel and shared our experiences with anyone who wanted to listen. I wanted to share my knowledge with others and learn more about how the body works. I tried to learn more about her syndrome, mostly to prevent anything like this from happening again. The syndrome itself didn't scare me—what did scare me was that the doctors who were supposed to be knowledgeable of the human body never looked at Trina as being anything but her syndrome. This may sound harsh, but it was reality.

Over time we just got on with life; her brother and sister felt that they could move on with their lives and that their sister was going to be fine. It was hard to see them go; they both moved and went to explore their lives in other parts of the province. We were very close and talked on the phone lots. Trina missed them so much; she would pick a piece of clothing from their rooms and wear it. After they moved she would look out the window and ask for them, or when we went out she would notice we were by their old homes and think we were going to visit.

Trina looked amazing; she had a sparkle in her eyes and a smile on her face. She was always a social butterfly, but now there was no stopping her. She started to swim again and enjoyed going for long walks. Sometimes she would just stand on the sidewalk and watch the cars go by. I often wondered what she was thinking about. I wondered how it would be to get inside her head and hear her thoughts. It would make me smile, remembering the dream I had about being inside her head. That dream saved her life; I know it as sure as I know that Trina picked our family to be with her on this Earth. I had a purpose that was like no other. School was wonderful for her; the life skills class brought out Trina's best. She loved going there and had a "big buddy."

The most amazing thing (well one of the most) was that her seizures stopped. Stopped completely! It was truly a miracle. Our lives changed. Except for her shot, no more doctors. No more pain and no more seizures. We didn't have to go to the hospital all the time; I didn't stay up all night and help her get through the pain. I didn't have a neurologist telling me that I was wrong for not having her on medication. This meant that I was right all along about all the medication not helping. If I had left her on medication that her body didn't need she definitely would not have been as healthy as she was and she would not have had the fight for life in her like she had. I could hug her and she would give me back the biggest hug back. She would touch my face when we lay together to watch her favorite shows. We would put on the stereo and we would dance together and laugh. Meals were once again with all of us sitting at the table, not me sitting on the couch spoon-feeding her because she couldn't feed herself. She would recognize people that she had met and or took care of her at school. Everything was great. This all happened before the Christmas of 2001. She was 17 years old. If there was ever a family that had something to be grateful for it was ours.

Our lives were filled with happiness and fun times. We once again went tobogganing and quading. We would have skidoos out in the bush with campfires, music, and a whole lot of laughing and just enjoying life. Spending time with friends was always something we enjoyed as a family and now we were going with the gang. The rest of the school year was amazing. Trina did so well in her new class—not once did I have to pick her up because she was sick or seizing. The calm that was in her, well you can imagine being in excruciating pain and still trying to function and learn. Now her brain was healthy, which allowed her to learn and retain.

Trina progressed every day. Her teachers couldn't believe she was the same child that they had either heard about in the school system or had taught before. The school year went by quickly and summer was upon us. She had a great summer— swimming in the pool, jumping on the trampoline. Her fear of the water was gone and she was swimming and wanting to jump off the diving board or just float in the water without a care in the world. She really didn't have a care then; Trina just loved to be alive. We took care of all her needs and made sure she was safe and had everything her little heart wanted. She was so easy to please and enjoyed the simple things in life. There was never a need to discipline Trina; she was not a child that understood the negative aspects of this world.

Denise F. Loewen

To be truly grateful for the little things in life is an understatement of what Trina's pain had taught us as a family. Every time she had the littlest accomplishment we would celebrate. I remember one time when I had taken her to a doctor's appointment for her vitamin B12 shot. I was telling him how great everything was and the progress that Trina was making. I guess I was a little emotional because he started to laugh and said our family sure knew how to be grateful for things so many others take for granted. I remember feeling great about what he said and took it as one of the best compliments I had received in a very long time. I guess I was still worn out from fighting with doctors who wanted me to feel less than that. It was so nice to hear that we were on the right track and enjoying life for real. Trina did that for us—she made us see the good in people and she taught us how to forgive. Living everyday to its fullest was how Trina lived.

Sadness still fills my heart some days. I just couldn't understand why she had to go through so much pain and be so misunderstood. I had spent so much time in our family doctor's office. One thing that was there that I'd read a thousand times while waiting in the waiting room was a saying that read:

WHEN YOU CAN'T CHANGE THE DIRECTION OF THE WIND, JUST ADJUST YOUR SAILS

I knew I couldn't change the path that Trina had chosen to take on her journey here on Earth. I certainly had to adjust my sails to go with the flow of her path. I had decided to learn how to give her the vitamin B12 shots myself. It just seemed to make sense, to give them to her at home instead of driving to the doctor's office twice a week. It didn't take me long to learn, and Trina didn't have to miss school. I think she missed seeing the doctor though—she still asked for him often. I would take her in to see him, just to thank him and show him how wonderful she was. He always got a big hug from her. She knew who was on her side.

Denise F. Loewen

Respect is a Two-Way Street—
If You Want It You Have to Give It

Something was wrong. Trina hadn't had any seizures and we hadn't been to the hospital for a long time. Then, almost exactly one year to the day that her seizures stopped from the vitamin B12, she had a seizure. I knew that she seizure from pain, so I thought maybe a headache was causing it.

Trina's pain tolerance was high; she had to be in a lot of pain before she would show any signs. Here is an example of how high it was: I was doing the dishes—Trina was almost 10 years old. The kids were playing outside in the back yard. It was a beautiful day. Trina came into the house to get a drink of cold water. (That's how she asked for water, "Cold, cold water." I got her a glass of water and when I bent down to give it to her I noticed there was blood all over the floor. I couldn't find any cuts on her, but it was coming from somewhere. I picked her up and put her on a chair to examine her closer. It was coming from her the bottom of her foot. She had stepped on a piece of glass and it was still in her foot. It was big, sticking in her foot about a half-inch or more. I called the other kids in to help me hold her still so I could take it out. She was upset and just kept saying she wanted to go jump—jumping on the trampoline was her favorite thing to do then. I pulled

155

out the glass, wrapped her foot in gauze, put some socks on her, and away she went to play outside. She didn't jump but she went out with the other kids without even a limp. That's just one story of many. I always had to keep an eye on her because she didn't seem to feel pain like you or I would. The pain tolerance has seemed to become more normal. If she stubbed her toe or banged her head she would say, "Ouch." But it had to be pretty hard.

I let the teachers know at school that she had a seizure and asked them to keep an eye on her and let me know if they noticed anything different about her behavior. They were very close to her and would notice even small things. Over a period of a few months things seemed off for her. She would stomp her feet on the floor and lean forward for a few seconds and then continue on her way. This would happen a couple times a day at first. Slowly, over the next few months, things seemed to get worse for her. We checked her B12 levels and all was good with that. Once again we were at the doctor's more and more, talking about the changes.

I started to notice that she would double over when she yelled, so this to me meant she had a stomachache. She wanted to eat more than she usually did—it was almost like I couldn't fill her up. With the pain came seizures that sent her to the hospital. Her blood pressure would drop and I'd have to call the ambulance. Again I was treated like I didn't know anything about my own child. If they couldn't get her seizures to stop a neurologist would be called.

Well, here went again about the seizure medications. I was stronger this time and stood up for her when new medications were brought up. I knew that Trina was in pain. When we were at the hospital I would tell them that she has a stomachache, and how she had been acting before we came. They

Denise F. Loewen

would take x-rays and find that her intestines were full of gas and that's why she had a stomachache. I didn't know a lot about the intestines so now I had something new to research. I learned about what foods gave you gas and I learned a whole lot about a stretched intestine. I knew this could be an issue for her because she'd had that bowel blockage when she was around eight years old. There was a lot to learn, but I needed to so I knew what I was talking about when I was confronted about her seizures. I learned about the gas medications that would help with gas build up, and about the foods that your body produces more gases from. I started to give Trina Tums and Gas-x to help relieve some of the pain. This did seem to help at the beginning, but as time went on it seemed like she needed more and more. I did not feel comfortable with this at all. I began to read about different diets and how they can help with the stomach digestion.

Our family doctor set up an appointment to see a gastroenterologist, a stomach specialist. The first time we talked about diet and that I could see a nutritionist to help with Trina's diet. We disused the pain that she was in and that it was causing her to seizure. I did think that I was able to keep her from some pain by feeding her bland foods. I agreed to see a nutritionist; I could use all the help and knowledge I could get. Most of the information that I learned there I had learned from reading and finding information on my own. But I truly believe if you already know 99 per cent of what you're learning and you only learn one new thing, it was definitely worth your time. It was extremely important to keep her bowels clean so the stretched part of her intestine could heal. It can heal, but it takes years, but Trina had been doing fine until now. I did learn that it is important not to eat foods with seeds in them. These seeds can collect in the bowel pockets and cause extreme pain. So with the bland foods and no seeds, Trina should have started to feel better. Some days she was not too bad and didn't really complain and then the next day she would be delirious with pain. I spent hours massaging her tummy for her, trying to release the gas build up.

By May of her graduation year once again I had to take her out of school. Because she enjoyed school so much, we tried hard to keep her going. The pain got worse and the length of time that she was in pain brought on seizures so strong that she couldn't function at school. She slept a lot from the seizing. The day of graduation pictures her teachers wanted me to bring her so she would have them. I thought we were going to make it, she was all dressed and we were almost out the door when she lay down on the couch and had a full grand mal seizure. So instead of getting grad pictures she ended up in the hospital getting x-rays. Once again her stomach was full of gas. There was no reason for this; she was eating healthy foods. I couldn't figure it out. To try and stop her seizures, the valproic acid that she was given before her B12 shots came back into play. I knew I had to have something to give her so I didn't have to bring her to the hospital all the time. This did help with her seizures, but not her pain. To get them to understand more about the fact that she was in pain, I would take her to the hospital before she started seizing. This was not fun and I hated doing this to Trina. When we went for the stomach pain I would drive her; if she was seizing I would call an ambulance. She was treated totally differently when I took her myself. I will explain to you in detail this one time and then from there you can imagine how things went down.

Trina had been sick all night, up screaming and trying to run out of the house. I tried to help her go to the bathroom and release some of her gas pain. Nothing worked.

She wouldn't eat or drink. She would sit on the toilet and pinch her tummy and yell. I had done all I could and knew we needed to go to the hospital. I drove her there; she was screaming and couldn't sit. I walked her up and down the hallway at the hospital. I tried to put her in a wheelchair so I could push her as I thought this might help. She was having no part of that. She needed to walk. I would get her to sit for a few minutes and then she'd need to get up and walk. I tried so hard to keep her quiet, but she couldn't do it. We were there for 11 hours walking, and people who were already angry before they got to the hospital would tell her to shut the f— up. They scared me. I couldn't do anything about it. Every time I would ask them to please get her in to see a doctor, they would just say, "Soon." Other people were ahead of her because she was not considered an emergency. I was so exhausted I could hardly stand up myself. Trina was starting to drag her left foot and buckle over from the pain, but still she couldn't sit down for any length of time. People came and went and nobody called her in.

By morning I was so tired and mad I wanted to throw up. I was sick for my daughter for being treated that way. I took her home. She didn't get to see a doctor; I could hardly drive with her. She kept taking off her seat belt and screaming. I finally got home with her and called our family doctor and told him what had happened to us and how she had been treated. I received a phone call from the hospital a few minutes later; they apologized and said for me to bring her back and they would get her in right away. I did take her back and they did see her. Her poor little stomach was so full of gas. I kept asking them what would cause her to have so much gas as she hadn't eaten anything that should cause it. They gave her some Adivan to calm her down and with massage on her tummy she slept she started to pass the gas. Then she slept and I took her home. After that visit I did everything I could to not have to take her back unless there was nothing else I could do. No one should ever be treated like that. Because Trina couldn't talk and say what was wrong and she was mentally challenged they just assumed that she behaved like that all the time. I tried to tell them she didn't but no one would listen to me. We did get treated much better after that visit, I'm sure thanks to her doctor.

The gas medicines were not working any more. Trina seemed to be trying to make herself feel better. She would eat soap—I mean bars of soap. I had to stop buying bars and only had liquid. Our doctor explained that babies will do that as a natural cleanser. Trina was 20 years old. She was trying to cleanse her own tummy. She started to eat and swallow things that were not food. She had never done anything like this before, not even as a baby. This was just beyond what I could ever have imagined. The seizures got worse—nothing was making her feel better. There was a medication for irritable bowel syndrome that was worth trying. I know it was hard to tell because Trina couldn't talk, but the gas build up was one of symptom of this syndrome. Our family doctor put her on a medication for this called Zelnorm. It seemed to help. She was able to go to the bathroom; it gave her diarrhea but that helped release her gas. With the reduction in her pain the seizures were happening less often. They were still too frequent for her to go back to school. She had missed the end of her last year and everyone was very sad about that. She'd had such a great year until this all began. It felt like going back in time, I had to once again argue with the professionals over and over about how this had nothing to do with her 3p minus syndrome. I'm not sure why this was such a big issue

Denise F. Loewen

for the specialists; all her life I had to fight with them to get them to listen to me, but here we were again. I was surprised; I had been right every other time she had been sick in her life. I felt that I had earned their respect.

Life really should not be that hard. Trina was such an amazing person and now was the oldest child with her syndrome. You would think that because she had surpassed all of what was expected of her that she would be treated even a little bit special. I felt that because she had lived longer and really had always been extremely healthy I would have been listened to more carefully. But instead I got, "Well, you should be grateful Trina lived as long as she did." Don't get me wrong. I was very grateful that she was still with me. What I was not grateful for was the fact that she had been in pain most of her life and needless pain at that.

I still had faith and hope that all would be okay. I would pray and be grateful for every day that we had together. I promised her every day that I would make her better. I would make appointments for her just to talk to her doctors to brainstorm and share my ideas with them. Most of the time I would leave the office feeling frustrated and unheard. Some might think that it was time to give up and accept what the doctors were saying, but I couldn't. Something in Trina's face and eyes when she looked at me told me there was a problem that needed attention and that I needed to take a deep breath and believe in myself and her. I was not the type of person to roll over and let others tell me what I should think, and this was not the time to start. I needed to continue learning everything I could about the digestive system. When the nutritionist would ask me about her diet and share her information with me about gluten and foods that could irritate the stomach or the bowels, I would learn about it. I started by putting her on different diets to see if anything would change. Sometimes it would seem like some things were working. Trina would have good days and then really bad days. This went on for months and then another year had gone by.

Nothing changed. Our visits to the hospital were always the same. She would have seizures, we would have to go in, they would take blood work, and they would find nothing wrong. Then it was x-rays and always back to her syndrome and how I needed to feed her better. There was nothing they could do for her; I was given a choice to leave her there or take her home. I always took her home with me. No one was going to have my daughter for any reason.

I was left with no answers and a bad feeling in my stomach. When would they get it? The medication that she was given for her seizures were Adivan and valproic acid. As time went on these were increased to help stop her from seizing. Nothing took her seizures away completely; they would just slow down for a while. These medications also slowed down the rest of her body. This was just another reason they had to use for her body shutting down.

I can't ever remember feeling that they were right, not ever. I would keep trying and not give up. I went to the extreme I guess; I was tired of her diet being the blame for her gas pain. I put her back on baby food. None of the diets I had tried worked so what else was there to do but to start over as if she were a baby? By dong this I would be able to tell if any one food was the cause. Starting with rice pablum, I added one food at a time. I did this for months, without much success.

Trina had lost the use of her right side by then and she couldn't do anything by herself. This was very frustrating for her as she had always been so independent. She couldn't

Denise F. Loewen

feed herself or walk on her own. Her right arm and leg did not have any strength any more. Trina didn't complain about the change in her diet. She not only lost the use of her body, but she also lost her speech. She no longer yelled in pain or walked for hours on end. She was getting sicker as the months went on. It seems impossible that it went on for so long, but it did.

The visits to the hospital never changed. What did change was I refused to have the neurologist that she had been seeing since she was six years old be called in to assess her when we were there. This didn't fit well with the staff, but I was at the point of not caring what any one else thought anymore. I knew by then that if something was not done for Trina soon, we were going to lose her. I asked for a different neurologist but there was a waiting period of eight months to see her. For me it was worth it. I still knew that being respectful to others is the way to get respect, but my Dad used to say to us when we were kids that if you have nothing nice to say don't say anything at all. The only way I knew I could follow his wise words of wisdom was to not let her be seen by someone that had no interest in finding out what was making my daughter so sick. I don't say this to be unkind; I'm telling you this because it's the only way I knew how to stay strong at this point in Trina's life. Finding out what was wrong meant life or death for her. Writing these words makes me feel sick even today.

THERE IS NO LOVE LIKE A MOTHERS LOVE

The time seemed like it was standing still and yet the days were going by so fast I don't know where they went. Birthdays had come and gone, grandchildren were born. (Trina became an auntie.) The little ones loved Trina so much they would sit with her and look at books with her. We tried so hard to go on like a normal family. I watched shows like House and any other doctor show I could. I remember thinking we need a doctor like House to come into our lives. The movie As Good As It Gets was another one that I watched and cried wishing that would happen for us. Sleep was a luxury; it was hard to close off the voice in my head praying that something would break and we would find out what was happening. I would take Trina for drives—walking was too hard for her and she hated sitting in a wheel chair. It was a fight every time I tried to get her in one. This just told me that she wasn't giving up and it was her way of telling me not to. She would pull my face to her face and look in my eyes with a look of pleading, the energy from her was saying, "Please don't listen to them, Mom. I am sick." While driving I would beg God to help me. Sometimes I would let him know that it was all beyond me. I didn't know what he wanted me to do and I would try and relax and give it back to the Earth. This would help sometimes. We would go home and I would continue to love her and take care of her as best I could. I tried not to think that my best was not going to be good enough. I promised over and over again that I would figure it out and that she would be able to live without pain. That's all I ever wanted for her: to live and love living. I really didn't think I was asking for too much.

I was trying not to take all of this personally, but it was getting really hard not too. Once again there were no answers and I was on my own to do the research. I certainly wasn't a doctor, but I sure felt like I had earned the name sometimes. As I said before, being at the hospital with Trina was harder than anything. When you are there you automatically

Denise F. Loewen

have some hope that this time, yep, this time they will do something. They can't just let her die. I couldn't increase her seizure medication any more, and there weren't any out there that we hadn't tried.

Once again we were back in the hospital. I knew we had to be there. She was too sick for me to have at home by myself, but calling the ambulance was so hard for me to do. I had been keeping her as healthy as I could; this meant feeding her and giving her liquid with an eyedropper. This was what I did all day long. I learned how to take her blood pressure and knew when I had to call and have her taken to the hospital. The saddest part about this is that I had to wait until she was so sick that I was scared before I called the ambulance. If I didn't, I knew they wouldn't even try to do anything for her.

I knew in my heart that this time all was beyond me. She needed to be on an intravenous drip to keep her from being dehydrated; she had lost the use of her whole right side and it was not coming back. I knew this time I would not have a choice as to who was going to be her neurologist this time— whoever was on call was who would see her.

Trina's sister had once again moved back to be closer to her little sister. I couldn't have taken care of her for as long as I did without her help. Her brother was living out of town, but was always as close as he could be by phone. He knew how sick she was and called often. Everyone was worried about her—that went without saying. All the kids who lived with us throughout the years were all very close to her and loved her very much. I had been talking to her all the way to the hospital, telling her it was going to be okay. I would make them treat her the way she should be treated. The ambulance attendants were always very nice and would ask questions about her. Most of them had gotten to know us very well and just couldn't believe our story. They always wished us luck before they had to leave us. Trina left a soft spot in their hearts every time. There is so much more I could tell you, but I think the important part of this story is what you need to hear next.

Once in the hospital Trina got in right away because this time she was seizing one after another and her blood pressure was very low. The nurses are and always were very caring and gentle with her. They also understood that I needed to do a lot of her care while being there. There were certain ways to do things with Trina that made her more comfortable, and she only trusted me. I was part of that team and they always seemed to be thankful that I was there with her. I knew a neurologist would be called almost immediately. There was no more fight in her as she lay there not making a sound. I could tell this was more serious than all the other times over the last few years—the faces of the staff showed that. They knew Trina had a fighting spirit in her that had gone. The neurologist was called and God was with us that night—it was the neurologist that we had been on the wait list to see for months. When I saw her I just looked up and said, "Thank you, thank you." I was the most relief I had felt in years.

It took her a long time to come in and see Trina, but when she did she had read her chart and knew things that I had forgotten. She asked me questions about Trina's birth and her younger years. I couldn't believe it. She spent a long time getting information from me and really seemed to care about the outcome. She didn't make me feel ridiculous about wanting my daughter to get better. I told her about the 3p minus syndrome and explained that even though Trina had been diagnosed with this, it was not why she was sick. This was an illness, not the end of her time. I tried hard to keep

Denise F. Loewen

my voice calm and not seem like a crazy parent who didn't have concrete information. We talked about all the diets I had put her on and why I did. When she brought up the foods that maybe she shouldn't eat I was ready. I told her I had put Trina on baby food months before and it had made little difference. She was pleased that we didn't have to start there, as that part had already been looked at.

The other part of Trina's information that she didn't understand was why a person that had so many seizures was not on seizure medication. I knew this was coming and I was ready for that question. It was one that I had been fighting about for a long time. We went over all the medications she had been put on and what side affects she suffered from. The one that was in her chart that I still can't believe was in there was the medication that her pediatrician had put her on when she was young. As I wrote about earlier on, he had put her on medication and she was like a zombie. Well, what he had put in her chart as the reason I wanted her off those medications was because she was losing a lot of hair. There was it no mention of her being over-sedated and without any quality of life. I was speechless. I didn't know how to respond to that. So I didn't. I didn't go on and on about how he almost killed her and had never done anything to improve her health. Even though that's what I felt like saying, I kept my mouth shut and took over the conversation. There was no need to go into her past any further. Her suffering from right then at that very minute had nothing to do with her syndrome or seizures. I very kindly said to her, "Look I know that Trina is in extreme pain. Her seizures come from pain. I also know that her pain is in her stomach area." I showed her on Trina where I felt her pain was. She listened to me now and really seemed to be hearing what I was saying. I felt that maybe she would help her instead of turning her illness onto me. When I was done explaining what I needed her to hear, I said, "If you can get rid of her pain, I know it's in her stomach, and if she is still having seizures I'll put her on any seizure medication you want me to." I also told her with the pain she was in there no seizure medication was going to stop her from seizing. We left it at that. She thanked me and left the little room that we were in. I sat beside Trina and talked to her and prayed that I had been heard.

Soon things started to happen. First there was a lot of blood work done. Then after that the nurses came in and started to get Trina ready to collect urine. This was difficult because she was pretty much comatose. I helped them take a urine sample and then we had to wait for some test results to come back. While we were waiting for those a nurse came in and told me they were taking Trina for an ultrasound. I was shocked. This was the first time anyone had taken a real interest at what I was saying. The only tests that were ever done were x-rays. All they ever showed was the gas build up that she was suffering from. I wish now that I had studied the different kinds of tests done by machines such as x-rays, ultrasounds and cat scans. I had heard of all of them, but never really understood what each one did and what they were used for.

They took Trina for the ultrasound and I went with her, of course. Nothing was done without me by her side. While we were in the room to start the ultrasound, Trina was very uncomfortable. It took me awhile to get her to relax so they could start. With this done, the ultrasound began. The technician was talking to us. She was very gentle and patient with Trina. It took a little longer than it would for someone else, but she talked to me and asked me questions about what had

Denise F. Loewen

been happening with her. I told her about Trina's stomach pain and all the x-rays we'd had done and how nothing ever showed up but gas. I also told her about the diets I had put Trina on and that I'd had very little luck with any of them. I was trying so hard not to cry, but was hard. Sometimes, once you start it seems like you will never stop. She was wonderful—listening and very caring. While I was babbling about how horrible the last few years have been for her she looks at me and said, "Honey, you don't have to worry anymore. It has never been anything you were doing wrong. And Trina won't have to go on any more of those diets." I wondered what she was talking about and asked her what she saw. Of course, she couldn't tell me anything, but she said just to wait there with Trina. With that she left the room to go find the doctor.

God Was Listening

I didn't know what to think. It sounded like the ultrasound technician found something and that Trina was going to be alright. I hugged Trina and tried to get her to stay on the bed. It seemed like forever before she came back. She did a little bit more with the camera, taking a lot of pictures. I tried to make some sense out of the pictures I could see on the screen, but I didn't know what to look for. I knew she couldn't tell me any more, but when she was done she wished us luck. I had a great deal of hope as we left that little room and Trina was wheeled back into the emergency room. We waited there for the doctor to come and talk to me and explain what had been found and if it was fixable. I say fixable because for the past years as I was trying to get someone to believe me, I was told over and over that Trina was not fixable and I had to accept how she was. One of the nurses came and talked with me and told me that the doctor would be in shortly to see Trina.

It felt like a lifetime, but finally she came in to tell me what had been found with the ultrasound. It was her gall bladder. Her gall bladder was so rotten that it had turned to sludge— Trina would have to have emergency surgery to immediately remove it.

I was so relieved that what she found wrong with Trina was fixable, and once again she would be fine. I immediately called her brother and sister to tell them the news. They couldn't believe it. Finally, after four years of their sister being so sick, some one listened and instead of shrugging me off as an over-protective mother.

There was more information that was very difficult to comprehend; because Trina's gall bladder was so rotten there was a chance that they would not be able to reattach the tubes to bypass the gall bladder. Hearing this made me scared once again. Trina's sister was now living in town, but her brother was hours away. They felt that it would be good to wait to do the surgery till her brother could get a flight home. This was to prepare for the worst: Trina not making it through the surgery. He came home on the next flight and the surgery was done the next morning.

Trina had lived through so many things that should have taken her from us, but she was still here. We knew the fight she had in her and we prayed for the best: to have her back with us so my promise to her could be fulfilled. I didn't want her last years on this Earth to be of extreme pain and misunderstanding.

It felt like a lifetime passed as we sat in the waiting room while Trina was in surgery. We sat and we paced. It was hard to talk about anything—it seemed that breathing was all we could do. The kids kept telling me she would be okay. As much as I wanted to believe it, I also knew how sick she had been and for how long. Could she bounce back again like she did after getting her vitamin B12 shots? It just didn't seem possible for one beautiful little soul to live with so much pain and still fight to be with us.

Denise F. Loewen

It was finally over—the surgeon came and told us she did great. They were able to reattach the tubes and he felt that she would heal. I was then allowed to go into the recovery room with her—that's a great thing about the hospital—they realized Trina needed me with her always. She did much better if she saw my face when she came out of the anesthetic. She was truly amazing. It didn't take her to long to wake up and before I knew it we were back in her hospital room.

Trina slept most of the day. The rest of us sat nearby and watched her sleep. There were lots of smiles between us; it was almost like being in another time, really. It was so incredible that she once again survived an illness that surely should have ended her life. I kept thinking to myself; I knew it I was right and the fight that I went through everyday to get someone to listen to me was worth every second. Trina rested well throughout the night. In the morning she woke up with me right beside her. She had intravenous tubes attached still in and did not like it. When she became wide awake she asked for toast and eggs. I knew she would be fine. She was already talking and trying to get out of bed. She hadn't done this for a long time. The kids had gone out and when they returned to the hospital they couldn't believe how spry she was.

It had been a long couple of years. Not just days or weeks—it had been years since she had been without pain. The little bit of pain she was probably feeling from the surgery was not even affecting her. She had some breakfast and wanted to get out of bed and walk around, so that's what we did. She headed straight for the exit door, ready to go home. The nurses were all very excited for her and happy to see her energy and personality were back in full swing. It always amazed me at how fast she bounced back after being ill for so long. Once she had eaten and gone to the bathroom they took out the intravenous tubes. This gave her much more freedom and there was no stopping her then.

We spent one more night in the hospital and the next day she was allowed to go home. Well there was a celebration to be had. There were lots of hugs and kisses as well as tears of joy for weeks to come. To have Trina home again healthy was something that brought back our faith in the world. Our family grew closer, if that was even possible.

Trina very quickly got the strength back in her legs. A few days of not having those nasty seizures was all it took. She had lost a lot of weight over the past few years and I can't tell you how nice it was to not have to feed her baby food anymore. Increasing her foods had to be done slowly, and now I had to learn about the function of the gall bladder and how her body would work without one. Like I've said over and over, knowledge is the way to go. There was so much to learn—and the more I did learn the angrier I became knowing how much pain she was really in all that time. Now I had to reroute that negative anger and try to make it into something positive. Trina needed me as much then as she did when she was sick. I had to work with her to get her body functioning well. The only way she could move ahead was if I was in a good frame of mind. It was not easy putting all those feelings of anger aside, but for her I did it and it made me a better person because of it.

YOU CAN'T ENJOY THE PRESENT
AND THE FUTURE WITH ANGER IN
YOUR HEART FROM THE PAST

Denise F. Loewen

That was a new chapter in my education and I felt good about winning that battle for her. Once again it was proved that her seizures were caused by pain. It was not hard for her to start doing all the things she enjoyed once again. Our family was bonded and I'm sure she was the glue that held it all together. Trina's brother moved back home shortly after her surgery. It was a very close call—we had almost lost her and being so far away and not being able to be with her as much as possible was a worry that he didn't want.

Many of her sisters and brothers came home to see her. She was always in their hearts. Trina's sister stayed close and helped me daily. Trina was able to spend much needed time with her nieces and nephew. They loved their Auntie Trina so much. They were the best therapy she could ever have. They made her laugh and smile. There was lots of love in her life. It's something we all need.

Back in Heaven

TRINA: Hi God. I'm back. What happened? I thought I was going to be down on Earth longer than I was.

GOD: Hi my Angel, It's so nice to see your smile. I needed you back here with me. Did you learn all you wanted to down there?

TRINA: Oh yes, and more. I was right about the family I chose. They were kind and loving. They accepted me for everything I was.

GOD: You look even brighter this time. Is it possible that you gained something from your family also?

TRINA: The faith and hope that they shared was amazing and they embraced me with all the strength and love I've ever experienced. It's healing to go back there sometimes—it fills my soul. I do feel brighter. I want to be so bright that even though I'm not with them in body, they will always feel the light of my spirit with them.

GOD: You are a very wise and thoughtful angel. This is why I let you chose when you wanted to go and experience the human mind. Only you know when you're ready and I trust that you will fill all the hearts that you connect with. I was so proud of how you communicated your inner thoughts with your chosen mother on Earth. You have made her a stronger soul and your love flows from her to all those she touches.

TRINA: Thank you. I am grateful for your kind words. I am strong and I know that when I'm down there you are always with me. But I still don't understand why you brought me back sooner than we had planned.

GOD: My darling little angel, your path was a powerful one. You endured more than even you had chosen. I brought back home when I did because you had reached and taught all the human souls you needed to. To have you suffer more would have broken the hearts of those in your family. Sometimes the best teaching is knowing when to let go.

TRINA: Thank you for taking care of my chosen family. I will wait now for them to come home to me. They will always know that I am with them in their hearts and souls.

Denise F. Loewen

Epilogue

It is now 2014. Our Trina has been back in Heaven for a little over two years now. I had thought of writing a book for years, long before we lost her. I always had so much to say about so many things—I didn't know how to start. After the loss of my baby girl I certainly had a lot of time to think about all the wonderful years we had her with us. Trina had touched so many people in her too-short life, and those she touched have her in their hearts forever. Many times people say to me that it was because of knowing Trina that they became better persons. The best ever is when something bad almost happens to someone and they feel Trina's presence and just know that she was there with them.

I know I wouldn't have been the mom I was and am without her in my life guiding me to forgive and be grateful for all the positive experiences that life offers us. I would like to take credit for Trina's sister and brother growing up to be the wonderful people they are, but most of the credit must go to Trina.

There have been many times throughout her life when I could have held on to anger— for her pain and those who didn't see her as we did. It was because of Trina's strength and love of life that I learned to leave the past behind and embrace the present and the future. Most of the wonderful friends that I have in my life I have because of Trina. We all became a team and continue to be there for each other even now. That I know I will never lose in my lifetime.

I truly believe that our special needs children come to the Earth to teach. They teach in ways that most of us can't even comprehend. All who have the privilege of learning from these children acknowledge that they changed their lives in a positive way, and think differently about gratitude and seeing the worth that each and every human being brings to this world. Even those who don't feel a connection to these special children, and may think that they didn't make an impact in their lives, are wrong. It may not be noticed at the time of being in the presence of these incredible children, but somewhere, sometime, it will happen, and they will have a change of heart in their future. Perhaps they won't even make the connection.

The reason why I needed to write this book was to continue the teachings that Trina had come here to do herself. I know this is what she would want to happen. There are so many people who struggle, as we did, with different systems. I hope all who read about Trina's life path will find strength and encouragement in it. As you read her story you will know that not giving up is the message I want you to get. When you have that feeling that something is not right, listen to it—it could mean life or death for yourself or for a loved one who cannot speak for themselves.

After Trina's last surgery she did extremely well. We had over ten years beyond what her lifespan was expected to be. Knowing that it was time to let her go was the hardest thing I've ever had to endure. In my heart I knew that she had done her teaching here on Earth and she was needed elsewhere.

Denise F. Loewen

I have cried a river while writing about the life of beautiful life of my baby girl. I have relived all those horrible times when I almost lost faith and didn't know how to have my voice—her voice—heard. Even though I have gone back in time remembering all the negativity she had to endure, I also was blessed by remembering all the joy and love that we lived and I wouldn't give up one second of our lives together; those experiences will follow me into my next path in this life. I have children and grandchildren, nieces and nephews, brothers and sisters, many friends and more life to live.

And I am grateful, so ever grateful, to have had the best teacher that there could ever be to have blessed my life.

CPSIA information can be obtained at www.ICGtesting.com
Printed in the USA
LVOW07*1936061114

412208LV00002B/3/P